Breathe

"This book is a gift to all who strive for better balance and wellbeing. Ela is uniquely qualified, drawing from her medical practice and her breathwork and holistic practices to bring invaluable insights and coping strategies for the full life we all aspire to have. Thank you Ela."

WENDY LUCAS-BULL, CHAIRMAN OF BARCLAYS AFRICA GROUP Ltd

"So much of what is happening on the planet, within and between societies, governments and cultures ... the wars and conflicts, the environmental problems, the breakdown of financial structures ... All this is a reflection, an extension, of our personal issues and challenges. With her book Breathe, Doctor Manga offers us a powerful and healthy alternative: become conscious of your natural life force energy, and learn to tap it and channel it in ways that are positive and sustainable. This book is meant for our times!"

DAN BRULÉ, BREATHWORK MASTER AND AUTHOR OF *JUST BREATHE*

Breathe

Strategising energy in the age of burnout

Dr Ela Manga

This book contains information that is intended to help readers be better-informed consumers of health care. It is presented as general advice on health care. Always consult your doctor for your individual needs.

No part of this book may be reproduced or transmitted in any form or by any means, electronic or mechanical, including photocopying, recording or by any information storage and retrieval system, without written permission from the author.

An earlier version of this book was published as *The Energy Code* in 2017.

First published by MFBooks Joburg, an imprint of Jacana Media (Pty) Ltd, in 2018

© Ela Manga, 2018

All rights reserved.

ISBN 978-0-620-86844-0

Cover design by Shawn Paikin
Set in Sabon 11/15pt

*I dedicate this book to The Great Mystery,
the ultimate source of all energy*

Contents

Foreword ix
Preface xiii

Introduction: Authentic energy 1
  1 The seven laws of authentic energy 9

Body Intelligence
  2 The intelligent pulse of life (IPOL) 25
  3 Eating for authentic energy 35
  4 Healthy hydration 48
  5 Sleep and rest 57
  6 Conscious breathing 66
  7 Exercise 81
  8 Tapping into nature 96

Mind Intelligence
  9 The effect of technology 107
10 Mindful living 120
11 Living in the present 133
12 The neurobiology of change 144
13 How belief systems affect energy 158

Heart Intelligence
14 Emotions and energy 171
15 Applying boundaries 184
16 Creating an energised life 192
17 Our story: Thanksgiving 202

Acknowledgements 204
Glossary of terms 206
References 209

Foreword

Suffering from stress and burnout has reached epidemic proportions in the world. If you make a list of the top ten health complaints that the average doctor hears every day, you will find that every one of them is linked to stress or burnout in some way.

Being busy and feeling exhausted has become 'normal'. In fact, most people, without realising it, have become addicted to the chemicals their body produces when they are stressed out. And many or most of our health problems are often caused by it!

The toll that stress and burnout has on our body–mind system, relationships, and performance and productivity simply cannot be ignored. We cannot afford to wait until we are incapacitated by stress and fatigue before we do something about it.

Enter Dr Ela Manga, and this important book. Ela's passion is in bringing mindfulness back into medicine and in inspiring conscious living as a way of restoring and supporting health and wellbeing.

This book is full of compelling, real-life stories about the effects of stress and is a treasure trove of practical tips for preventing and recovering from it. It is a perfect guide for anyone faced with the pressures of modern life who is open to an integrated and mindful approach to optimum wellness.

This book explains clearly what supports our energy, how

to recognise and manage the things that drain our energy, and shows us how to harness the stress response so that it works for us instead of against us. In short, this is a book about an exciting new approach to healthcare called 'energy management'.

As a starting point, Ela shares with us her own remarkable story. She teaches us the basic laws and principles of genuine or authentic energy. And throughout the book she lays the foundation and a path to living on natural or 'authentic' energy instead of the adrenalised energy that has become the norm.

She has created a collection of energy formulas that you can use to generate and sustain natural energy throughout your day. Many high performers are aware of their body's signals and have developed their own strategies to cope with stress. They know what to do to keep going. They know what supplements to take and what food to eat. They deal with their symptoms as they encounter them in a practical way. They exercise and do yoga. They have learned to cope with their energy rollercoasters. But in many ways, all these strategies only allow them to function at baseline. This book will take these high performers to a new level of health and wellbeing.

Ela encourages and supports people in re-evaluating old, established habits and patterns. She points out that it's not just what you do, but how you do it that is important. For example, she explains how an exercise regime may be working against us rather than for us, and how using exercise as a way to tune out or distract ourselves is actually counterproductive, and how by focusing on the external benefits, working out has the potential to do more harm than good.

Dr Manga offers some simple yet powerful ways to integrate what she calls recovery loops into our everyday lives. She describes how the brain is designed and how to use mindfulness to harness mental energy. She also explores ways to use technology to support rather than drain our energy.

Ela practises what she preaches. She maintains a busy private medical practice, does holistic consulting, writes articles for leading health magazines, does radio and television interviews, speaks at conferences, leads seminars and trainings, does research and supports community-based programmes. She spends time alone in nature, and she has learned to integrate her personal and professional life. She listens to her body and she makes use of heart intelligence. She paints, practises yoga, does business and enjoys a rich personal and family life.

She is a genuine student and teacher, devoted to a life in service to others. She radiates love and light, and that energy comes through her words in this book. Ela is also the only medical doctor in South Africa who is a certified Breathwork practitioner and trainer. She is making a real difference in the world, and this book is sure to make a real difference in your life.

This book is a gift to the world. In fact, I believe that this unique and groundbreaking work will do more to help you prevent and recover from stress and burnout than anything you have learned and anything that has been published to date.

Dan Brulé, author of *Just Breathe*
May 2017

Preface

I have an early memory of myself as a little girl sitting on my beloved grandfather's lap as he painted a floral border around every page of his handwritten memoirs. As a historian and writer, he spent many hours in his study compiling photographs and stories of the Gujarati community who were living in different parts of the world. His own story told of a young boy of 14 who had docked on the shores of South Africa after a long sea journey from India with his father in 1926. It was a time when many Indian tradesmen and artisans were making their way to South Africa to set up businesses. They settled in the coastal town of Port Elizabeth where he helped his father start a small shoe-repair business. His heart was set on becoming a doctor, but due to the lack of financial resources his dream lay barren. Instead, he channeled his energy and focus into his business, which grew to sustain his family and put two of his sons through medical school. His two older sons remained in the business, which by then had evolved into a men's clothing outfitter. One of those sons was my father, who died of a massive myocardial infarction. I was only three years old.

The story that unfolded subsequently is layered and tangled, but when I pause and look over my shoulder to gaze on my formative years, I see the golden threads from my heritage that I have woven into my life. Every tragedy, every loss, every relationship of my early years has deepened my capacity to feel and love. It has instigated a curious bewilderment of the bizarre and wonderful complexities of human nature. For loss and adversity, I am grateful. Because of it, I grab onto life earnestly and with deep regard. And because of it, I draw beautiful people into my life and never let them go, unless I know it's time. But it certainly was not all bleak. I was a child who was indulged with love and attention from my mother and extended family. I'm not quite sure if I inherited my mother's zest and tamed rebellious nature or whether she projected it onto me, but it's undeniably there.

In my early teenage years, I held onto the dream of leaving home and studying Indian classical dancing somewhere in India, but alas, it was brushed off as a fanciful teenage notion. My next choice for a career was journalism. Perhaps unconsciously, there was a restless curiosity even then, an instinct to get a handle on the mystery of the human condition through words and stories. But it was not to be. I was told that it was not a real career and certainly not a lucrative profession, so I dropped that idea too. Medicine was the more responsible choice. Coming from a family of medical professionals, I was strongly encouraged to pursue a career in the medical field, and I can't say that I protested too much. When I was 14, my beloved grandfather fell ill. Each day after school for about two months, I spent time nursing him and at the same time soaked up his wisdom and deepening grace. It was a profound time in my life that shaped some of my fundamental beliefs of life and death. It was also my first experience of healing.

There were aspects of studying medicine that I loved, the privilege of dissecting a human cadaver, the examination of bizarre specimens in the pathology lab and then seeing real-life pathology in the hospital wards. But unlike many other brilliant students in my class, I had to work really hard and spent many, many hours bent over my notes and textbooks. I never tolerated late nights and lack of sleep, which meant I was probably miserable and cranky a lot of the time. Looking back, my two years of internship and community service were probably the most challenging of my career, but it was this experience that informed the choices that later shaped my work. I experienced burnout first hand and the emotional numbness that came with desensitisation from over-exposure to suffering. I salute the thousands of doctors and nurses who tolerate and bear what I could not.

We need and expect our caregivers to operate at the highest level of skill and dedication, but often that is not easy. That's one of the big reasons I have written this book because I know that our carers, our change makers, our creatives, our entrepreneurs and our leaders need support. We need the tools to support ourselves in a world of constant demand.

After my hospital stint, I was given the opportunity to locum at a small GP practice, which I subsequently took over. Finally, I felt free. I could go home every night and sleep in my own warm bed. I didn't have a boss to answer to. I also had to quickly learn the ropes of running a practice and get my head around accounts, admin issues and medical aids. It was a sharp learning curve but I learned the basics of running a business, which stood me in good stead. My practice was situated in a densely populated, vibrant community of young families just starting out life, as I was. I met many fascinating people. Between coughs, colds, gastro-enteritis, urinary tract infections and headaches I was managing HIV, alcoholism, drug addiction, auto-immune conditions, depression, anxiety, schizophrenia, bipolar mood disorder and injuries from drunken brawls. One day a woman walking past my practice went into labour. Adrenalised energy kicked in, putting everything into sharp focus. I delivered the baby right in my rooms. I saw it all. It was wonderful for a while and very necessary for my growth as a doctor. But soon, as restlessness and frustration began to stir in me, I felt like I was skimming the surface of what was possible in terms of supporting sustainable wellness. I was treating symptoms in an automated way bound by protocols and on the information I was being fed by drug representatives. It was becoming very clear that I was treating the tip of the iceberg of the body-mind-heart system and that underlying the physical symptoms was something that ran deeper. I needed to understand how it all worked, what really caused illness and what I could do to work at THAT level. I went on an exploratory mission to find doctors who were practising in this way and courses to study that would support my understanding. But that was 10 years ago and I felt alone in the wilderness. There were not many doctors who practised holistically, but I did come across a doctor in Cape Town, Dr Bernard Brom, who at the time was the editor of a magazine called *Natural Medicine*. I bought every edition and devoured the articles. Dr Brom is one of my mentors and teachers who remains deeply committed to training many doctors in the field of integrated medicine.

One day, during this time of my quest, a woman entered my life who changed the course of it. When Marisa and I first met, it felt as if I was reunited with a long-lost sister I had always known. She was exactly my age and a social worker by training. At the time, she was running holistic spas, one in Johannesburg and another from her family home near the Cradle of Humankind. We found that we shared the same vision of holistic wellbeing and our conversations become the catalyst for breaking free from the way I had been practising. We spent hours over copious amounts of tea, making plans and visualising the healing centre we dreamed of creating. More than that, we developed a deep friendship that has endured so much change. For about a year, Marisa spent some time at my practice, offering counselling services for my patients. Every now and again, I would take a drive out to the country and spend time at her spa with her and her mom, Mary.

I clearly remember the morning of a day in 2006 when I made the decision to sell my practice. It was time to make our dreams a reality. It was a giddy time, full of dreams and possibilities. I had just trained in an energy healing modality called 'Body Talk' and had started to craft my own version of integrated medicine. During that year, she built a beautiful centre on the banks of the river on her family property and the two of us began to craft an integrated model of healing that combined our skills and created a space that supported conscious living. This sacred space continues to be a sanctuary for many and is where I still run my practice today. Over the next few years my medical practice and her counselling practice grew and evolved as did our combined methodologies and treatments. We designed 8–12 signature treatment programmes, which included yoga, massage and coaching. We deepened our exploration of mind-body medicine and sparked awareness in people to support their health in a more sustainable way. Our clients became partners in the creation of their health. However, we began to notice an alarming trend in the people we were working with. We found that these passionate people, individuals who were really making a difference in the world – entrepreneurs, human rights activists, NGO and healthcare workers, change makers, visionaries and artists, moms staying at home to raise future-fit children – were starting to lose their fire. They were burning out. It was showing up in various ways – emotionally and physiologically – in their relationships and at work. I noticed a common thread of physical symptoms playing out: chronic headaches, insomnia, hypertension, heartburn, hormonal imbalances, irritable bowel syndrome, musculoskeletal issues, allergies, even auto-immune disease and cancer. Burnout didn't happen suddenly; it crept up on them and, before they knew it, they felt disconnected from the passion that had defined them. We began to get really curious about this idea of 'energy', not in the new-age esoteric sense, but rather energy in terms of capacity and performance; what fuels it, what drains it, the principles that define it and how we can sustain, maximise and replenish it.

Then something interesting happened. In 2012, five years after the centre was established, Marisa was given the opportunity to head up a project at Deloitte Consulting South Africa, called the 'Energy Journey', which she very successfully used as an opportunity to put our methodologies to the test.

While she took this idea of energy to the corporate world, I remained focused on the individual. The very same energy patterns that I was seeing playing out in individuals, she was seeing on a macro level in teams and organisations; systems working in silos, disconnected and fragmented, resulting in disengagement and sub-optimum performance.

Working within a holistic framework offered a perspective that went beyond the idea of burnout as a psychological state or adrenal fatigue as a medical condition. I began to see the same pattern of energy playing out in all the patients and clients I was seeing, and even in myself. I faced the reality that most of us are, in fact, somewhere along the road to burnout, and that unless we understand the strain that modern life places on our energy system and address it appropriately, we are at risk of burnout becoming the epidemic of the modern digital age. It affects all of us and we have no choice but to begin to deepen our understanding of the way energy works.

One day, I was consulting with a woman who was very animated and energised. She spoke with wide-eyed passion, sitting on the edge of her chair, barely catching a breath between sentences. But she reported feeling trapped in her busyness and carried her wide eyes to bed. It occurred to me that the quality of her energy was adrenaline driven, different from a more focused calm energy that would have been more appropriate for the situation. For the following three years, I became a student of energy and a devotee of the life principles by which it is defined.

What you are about to read is a refined framework of the principles of energy shaped by my medical background, the study of the mind-body connection, yoga, natural medicine and the latest advances in neuroscience, but mostly by the stories and conversations that I have had with my friends and the hundreds of incredible people who I have had the privilege of sitting with in my consultation room. It's through their life stories that I have learned the most.

The characters in these stories are based on actual people I have worked with. (Names have been changed.) Some of the stories are true to life, while others are a few stories rolled into one. The characters are all based in Johannesburg, South Africa, a throbbing metropolis that is defined by its tenacity, creativity, fear, passion, growth and change – a cauldron of adrenalised energy. But at the same time, you will find that their stories are universal.

In many ways, I have written this book for myself, to try and make sense of what I have discovered on my journey and to guide my work going forward. While some of the information in this book is as ancient as the mountains, I offer you a perspective that comes from real-life stories and that is relevant, simple enough and sophisticated enough for modern times. I offer you *Breathe*.

INTRODUCTION

Authentic energy

If seen for what it is, burnout can be a catalyst for growth and change, and an opportunity to create a life that is authentically energised and meaningful.

Have you noticed how being busy and exhausted is becoming a normal part of our daily narrative?

Fatigue is a global crisis that is having a major impact on the health of our individual and collective systems. Chronic fatigue syndrome, adrenal fatigue and burnout are common terms, which attempt to classify sets of symptoms that are in fact varying expressions of the same personal energy crisis.

While we are undeniably becoming more aware of the link between stress and health, are we really doing anything to change the way we are supporting ourselves in a world that is just becoming more and more demanding and distracting? Or do we keep seeking relief in a pill, fulfillment in another job and peace in another city or country? Will we keep repeating the same patterns until a crisis demands that we manage our lives differently?

No matter where we live in the world, or no matter what form our particular stress takes, we cannot escape it. In some cases, the stressors that we face are very real, exerted by an extremely demanding environment. Some of them may even be life threatening.

In many other cases, the stress we experience is an internal process based on how we are thinking about and perceiving ourselves and the world. In most cases, it's a combination of the above. The point is that it's there. Our exposure to local and global news, job uncertainty, financial stress, managing a home and children, educating children, technostress, building businesses, dealing with personal loss, striving for meaning and success, losing weight, keeping fit and keeping sane are all part of what we deal with every single day. Even if we are doing the work we love, somewhere along the line, our natural energy becomes tangled in routine, processes and neglected feelings. Busyness becomes habitual, lack of sleep the norm. We become addicts of our own stress. And like any addiction, it becomes destructive.

Typically, any new journey, whether it be a new job or relationship, begins with excitement, passion, inspiration, hope and optimism, all of which are powerful sources of energy. Because our 'energy battery' is still full, we have more resilience in dealing with challenges. We feel like we have capacity to manage it and tenacity to push through it. We work hard, push long hours, thrive on the fast pace and experience the rush from the rush. We get things done, we move and groove as we single-pointedly drive ourselves towards our goals. The more our system adapts to the pace, the more adrenaline we need to feel the same high and exhilaration to which we have become accustomed. We start to look for the next fix, the next crisis, the next drama with more coffee, cigarettes, caffeinated drinks and sugar-laden food added to the mix. We become locked and tangled in the web of doing. We start living in the head. We disconnect from our physical bodies and other sources of energy, and allow little time for recovery and replenishment. The stress response, instead of being the energy-giving response it is designed to be, starts to turn against us, chipping away at our energy and disconnecting us from our other sources of energy, our physical bodies, feelings and emotions, nature and relationships. Early symptoms of burnout creep up on us gradually and insidiously, manifesting not just physically but also in our behaviours, interaction with others, ability to focus and capacity to feel.

We have moved far beyond the age of stress management. That is a concept more relevant for a bygone era. We are now living in a time that demands new strategies in order to thrive. Energy management is not a quick-fix approach or something that can be achieved with the flick of a switch. It requires an inner enquiry, a thorough examination of our habits, choices, relationships and the influence of our environment on our energy. But before we get into that, let's get underneath the science of how this incredible body-mind system is designed and how we are able to become architects of an upgraded version that supports our life, our passion and purpose.

Every living creature is designed to survive. Whether it is moss on a rock or a mighty hump-backed whale, survival is an innate state, a primal response. Survival requires adaptation, evolution, stealth strategies, camouflage, intelligence and resilience. Built into the design of this survival system is an ingenious neurobiological mechanism that primes and fuels energy when we need it and that restores, heals and replenishes our energy reserves when we don't. The efficiency and efficacy of this system is dependent on the interplay of these two 'energy' systems. The natural world is a pure expression of the ebb and flow of this rhythm.

Our evolution as humans is reflected most profoundly in the way the brain has adapted and evolved. It is both astonishing and perplexing what the human mind is capable of. By virtue of our intelligence, we have attempted to outsmart nature to the point that we have outsourced our brains to digital devices! We have come up with unfathomable inventions: we can grow organs, travel into deep space and digitally print practically anything. However, while our brain has sprouted new neural connections and our grey matter has bulked up, the optimum functioning of our body is still very much dependent on the ancient rhythm of energy and recovery. The link between the two is something that is required for the next leap in our evolution. That link is awareness.

But I'm getting ahead of myself. Let us systematically follow the neurological pathway of the stress experience. Through the

Breathe

Dr Ela Manga

ENERGY ZONE MAP ©

OPTIMUM ZONE
- Open breathing
- Connected to body's signals
- Quality sleep
- Healthy bowel habits
- Strong immune system
- Ability to relax
- Self aware / mindful
- Strong boundaries
- Emotionally intelligent
- Focused, self motivated
- Strong social connection
- Well rounded

DANGER ZONE
MORE WIRED THAN TIRED
- Rising cortisol levels
- Sleep disorders
- Bowel irregularities
- Muscle tension
- High BP
- Shallow breathing
- Overuse of stimulants / relaxants
- Weight gain / weight loss
- Difficulty switching off
- Scattered focus
- Irritability
- Anxiety

TIPPING POINT

BURNOUT ZONE
MORE TIRED THAN WIRED
- Dropping cortisol levels
- Constant fatigue
- Sleep not restorative
- Hormonal imbalances
- Brain fog
- Loss of focus / memory / concentration
- Apathy
- Loss of direction / passion / trust
- Weight gain / weight loss
- Loss of meaning
- Depression
- Difficulty to self motivate
- Disconnection from support network

Adrenal fatigue
Chronic illness
Suicidal thoughts

Recovery loops

SOURCE ENERGY Body / Mind / Heart } Intelligence

drelamanga.com

supersensitive functioning of our sensory system, anything that is perceived as stressful, threatening or dangerous sparks up electrical activity in the parts of the brain that regulate stress. Electrical energy transforms into chemical energy as the signals ripple down through the hypothalamus-pituitary-adrenal axis in the brain in milliseconds. A chemical cascade ensues. Adrenaline floods the system, locking onto the cells in our vital organs. The pulse quickens, the breathing rate increases, the pupils dilate, our hairs stand on end. Blood gets shunted away from the digestive system to the vital organs of the heart and lungs. The entire body-mind system either gets primed for action or shuts down to become invisible to the threat. But it doesn't end there; the next wave of the stress response follows. Cortisol is released from the outer layer of the adrenal glands to provide more sustained energy and to manage any possible injuries that could have occurred in the dangerous encounter. Cortisol activates glucose stores from the muscles and liver. It behaves as an anti-inflammatory in case of injury and an immune system suppressant to conserve resources.

This entire process is a powerful energiser, providing us with almost superhuman power and energy to deal with the situation at hand. It seems that the level of activation of this response is directly proportional to the perception of the level of danger.

Once the energy is activated and channeled into the appropriate form of action, the wave subsides, and the rest and recovery/ rest and digest mode kicks in. We heave a sigh of relief that we have survived. The blood and energy resources shift back to the digestive system. Digestive juices start to flow, cells regenerate and the immune system gets supported. We slow down as we recover, recuperate and regenerate.

A perfect system for a perfect world.

Where this system fails us is that even a perceived threat is dealt with as a real one, activating the very same stress response as an actual event. The very nature of our modern mind is to think up potentially stressful situations all day. The fact that we carry our work in our minds and its device extension means that we are chronically in a low-grade fight–flight mode.

The energy zone map on page 4 is a tool that I designed to create awareness of the big picture, the inter-relatedness between the typical physical, behavioural and emotional symptoms that we experience as our energy system starts getting disrupted and as we drift from optimum zone to danger zone and eventually to burnout zone. When we are in optimum zone, we experience a sense of authentic energy or calm vitality. We experience the full expression of natural energy or source energy that is within us and in nature. We are self-aware, able to self-care and have a regulatory balance of adrenalised energy through recovery loops or conscious activation of the relaxation response. The specialised terms used throughout the book are defined in the glossary on page 206.

Slowly, we unknowingly creep from the optimum zone where we are using the stress response efficiently into the danger zone where the adrenaline becomes addictive. We will know when we are there. The body will give us tell-tale signs. Constant high levels of adrenaline and cortisol in the system means that we will experience digestive niggles: heartburn, bloating, constipation, abdominal cramps. The immune system takes a knock as we become more susceptible to infections, allergies and autoimmune conditions. As we experience more glucose spikes we are more prone to insulin resistance and our weight creeps up as our thyroid hormones are less effective. The body morphs as our musculoskeletal system contracts causing tightness in the jaw, shoulders and hips. The part of the brain that regulates stress becomes activated, and we tend to feel more irritable, angry and cynical. We seem to switch off as the mind takes on a frenetic life of its own, recreating and pre-creating stressful scenarios. We stay trapped in this mode, waiting for the weekend, dazed by the mirage of the next goal, the next holiday, reaching for satellite dreams of happiness.

Some of us are able to stay in this zone for a lifetime, putting self-care measures in place occasionally. Others are not as lucky; a small event can be the trigger that tips us over the edge, taxing the adrenal glands to a point where they are not able to keep up with the demands of our lifestyle any longer. We find ourselves in the burnout zone. When we are here, it becomes more and more difficult to muster up the energy to get out of bed. We begin to drag ourselves through the day, need more stimulants to get going, more aids to wind down. Chemical imbalances become more deeply entrenched and the world feels grey.

If seen for what it is, burnout can be a catalyst for growth and change, and an opportunity to create a life that is authentically energised and meaningful. We can consciously change the architecture of our brain to bridge the gap between our primal responses and our new evolved minds. When we do this we can upgrade our software from being unconscious to conscious beings that use the aspects of modern life to dig deeply and take responsibility for our choices, health and lives.

It is the easiest and the most difficult thing to do: easy because it is so obvious and so basic; difficult because it takes time, constant effort and awareness to create new habits and behaviours.

The key to staying in the optimum zone is simply to activate recovery loops, consciously and deliberately activating the rest and recovery mode. Recovery is the new paradigm in peak performance and energy management. We have to retrain ourselves to relax in the eye of the storm. It's as simple as that. When we can do that, then we can adapt the stress response and channel it so that we can use it as the energy-giving response it is meant to be.

This is not an easy process. Habits, patterns and behaviour that feed our adrenalised state have become habitual and unconscious and require awareness and effort to unravel.

Throughout the book, I will talk about ways to activate recovery loops through our three fundamental channels of energy: the body, mind and heart.

We keep our energy battery full by constantly attending to key aspects of who we are and three interconnected systems: body, mind and heart. The physical body is the foundation of energy. And as we know, when life gets tough, physical care is the first thing we compromise. Our bodies, being forgiving, are able to handle a great deal through their innate intelligence before they start to complain. In this section, through some real stories, we will look at some simple ways to tweak your lifestyle to harness our physical energy formulas. We will draw on some ancient wisdom and cutting-edge research so that you are able to craft your own energy strategy. We will maximise our body intelligence.

Mastering our body intelligence will give us a head-start in our attempts to maximise our mind intelligence. In this section, we will delve into neuroscience and explore the art of mindfulness as the key skill to break out of energy-draining, reactive behaviour and patterns. When we can do that, we open the door to our most potent source of energy, our heart intelligence. Through heart intelligence we can live creatively, harness our passion using the energy of our feelings and emotions as fuel for a richer and more meaningful life.

The 'Energy Formula' that appears at the end of each chapter is a summary or formula that encapsulates the essence of that chapter. It is designed to enable you to apply the formula to access your own authentic energy in a way that is relevant for you.

Journey with me to the place of energy mastery as we share stories that will inspire and shape your understanding of the amazing creative being that you are and the ways in which you can access your own energy resources.

How to use this book

Breathe is not meant to be read cover to cover or skimmed over in one weekend. It is a companion for a journey of inner discovery and enquiry. Digest one chapter at a time, sequentially or even randomly. Reflect on it, have conversations about it, keep a notebook handy and practise the exercises. There are parts of this book that will entertain you and parts that will make you cry. There are some that might irritate you and some that may even inspire you. Feel it all. Through the characters, you will see yourself and feel solace in the knowledge that at the end of the day we are all the same, desiring and deserving the experience of living with true authentic energy.

CHAPTER 1

The seven laws of authentic energy

Energy is optimised when we work with our cycles and rhythms rather than against them.

> **JACK'S STORY: REBELS AND LAWS**
> **Name:** Jack Rourke
> **Age:** 30
> **Character traits:** Passion, courage, optimism
> **Life-changing experiences:** Living abroad, failure of first business
> **Stress catalysts in last two years:** Constant pressure of a rapidly expanding business
> **Stress indicators:** Constipation, recurrent upper respiratory tract infections
> **Presentation on energy zone map:** Danger zone

It is a clear winter's morning in Johannesburg. The sun ascends over the high-rises in the east and streams into Jack's Manhattan-style apartment in the city centre. He's been restless and half-awake since 3:30am. Ideas and plans for his next project filter into his dream state, blurring the edges between dreams and reality. His laptop lies open on the floor next to his bed. He reaches for it and begins his day. Emails land in the inboxes of his financial manager, architect, another developer in São Paulo, and in mine. He's rescheduling his weekly appointment with me. He's flying to Scandinavia to meet with a sought-after architect. Over 340 emails have suddenly arrived in his inbox from the night before. He'll deal with it later, after coffee. His throat feels dry. In fact, he usually feels dehydrated, but today all his airways feel dry and inflamed too. He can't afford to get ill now, especially with this upcoming trip. He slaps his laptop shut, swallows a green-and-red capsule and heads for the door, his unfussed chocolate hair still damp from the shower. He half trips down three flights of stairs, cursing the project manager. The lift still hasn't been fixed. That's the downside of living in the precinct that he's developing. He literally lives at work.

The hole-in-the-wall coffee shop has just unrolled its shutter. Jack is the first customer waiting for his regular order, a double espresso and bowl of muesli. He feels the familiar achy burn under his ribs. This is becoming a source of anxiety. He makes a note to discuss the issue in our next session. Moments later, he is joined by his sales manager. Next the Swiss artist arrives. He is erecting a sculpture on one of the rooftops. Both appear like thirsty beasts heading to the watering hole. The conversation becomes more animated as caffeine lights up their neural pathways. Jack forgets his sore throat and moody bowel and darts across the street to his first meeting with the mayor. By the time evening comes, he is flat on his back. His throat is on fire, there's a vice grip across his chest and his heart is pounding. He calls his mother.

Jack Rourke is young, curious and courageous. He is a visionary who brings his dreams to life with passion and tenacity. He's comfortable with risk and dares to be different. His mantra of 'screw normality' is reflected in obvious and subliminal ways throughout the inner-city precinct which he began to redevelop at the age of 26. Most thought he was reckless when he went into one of the most derelict parts of the Johannesburg city centre. He did it anyway.

He's an eternal optimist with the soul of a hippy and the mind of a maverick, driven by a vision of a conscious society based on community, collaboration, entrepreneurship and artistic expression.

Being the CEO of a rapidly expanding property development company and ambitious social entrepreneur demands that Jack be always on top of his game. His days are long and packed with meetings, interviews, and calls with his investors, architects and operational team. When he's not travelling, he starts his day before the world wakes. This is his time to dream and formulate his ideas into plans. There are unexpected moments when Jack looks through his office window across the rooftops of the precinct and is overcome with anxiety. The enormity of his job and the responsibility he feels for the people who have made this neighbourhood their home is overwhelming. These moments are rare but in the days preceding his first consultation with me, they had become more frequent than was comfortable for him. His usual optimism felt contaminated by anxiety. And anxiety pulled him into a downward spiral of despair and disillusionment.

It was at this point that I met Jack. His choice to see me was driven by his awareness that his physical and emotional health was taking strain. He was also curious about exploring a more unconventional and sustainable approach to managing his health and energy going forward.

Living in the precinct that he was developing meant that he was living and breathing his work every day with no respite. His analytical mind dissected every detail he observed while his creativity fed his dreams and visions. He needed to find a way to keep his fire burning without it burning out. For Jack, like many other entrepreneurs, there was no separation between life and work. In fact, his work was born from a desire to create a free, creative, urban lifestyle. What struck me most about him was his infectious optimism and passion for life. It was a rare experience to be with someone who embodied two very distinct qualities of energy at the same time. A certain quality of joyful energy shone through when he spoke of his greater vision, the community he was creating and the people who were part of it.

And yet his posture, breathing pattern and distractibility reflected a wired energy that for the purposes of our consultation was out of context. Jack was perturbed that he ticked so many of the boxes in danger zone on the energy zone map, but when I explained the symptoms in the context of the stress response, it made more sense. He acknowledged that his body had felt more knotted and tense in the preceding month and the episodes of heartburn were becoming a more frequent occurrence. An adrenalised energy state had become his new normal and was contaminating his natural energy. He couldn't deny that it was beginning to impinge on his work, relationships and health, and that continuing to live in this way was simply not sustainable.

To live with more authentic energy, a change of perspective was required. Jack was being challenged to redesign his lifestyle and design his working day to support his unique body type and energy cycles. But first, we had to explore some fundamental concepts. In order to master our energy system, it's helpful to understand the fundamental laws and principles that define them. We are part of nature and its rhythm and eternal cycle. We are born. We die. And no matter how sophisticated our technology, no matter how effective our medicine, we are governed by its laws. Working against nature's perfect design will inevitably get us into trouble. Burnout is simply a symptom of us living out of sync with who we truly are and our natural energy sources. If we are committed to living optimally and consciously, we have a responsibility to get right back to the basics, to understand the laws and principles of energy in the way that our forefathers did, the way the indigenous people did. We have a responsibility to innovate a new way of living that is relevant for modern times and yet honours the role of traditional wisdom. I am blessed to be working in an environment that supports my observation of nature's inner workings. Our greatest teachers and role models in energy mastery are those who live most intimately with nature and as natural beings. They remind us that the source of natural energy is right within and around us. We just need to find simple, modern and innovative ways to tap into it. Jack was ready to figure out how.

For Jack to manage his energy in a way that worked with his unique lifestyle and energy blueprint, he had to start by understanding the fundamental laws (see page 20) and how to apply them.

We began with the law of rhythms.

There is a universal pattern or rhythm of energy that we see from the microcosm to the macrocosm. We see it in the ebb and flow of ocean waves. It is evident in the cycle of seasons; the high-energy seasons of spring and summer and low-energy cycle of winter, the time of introspection and hibernation. It's evident in the lunar cycle; the high energy of full moon and low energy of the waning moon. We feel it in our biorhythms, circadian rhythms and menstrual cycle.

We experience it with every heartbeat and with each inhalation and exhalation. The very functioning of our cells depends on the oscillation of this energy. Our neurobiological system reflects this rhythm as the high-energy-giving 'stress response' governed by the sympathetic nervous system and the relaxation or the 'rest and digest' mode governed by the parasympathetic nervous system.

The high-energy state of the stress response (adrenalised energy) naturally drops into the recovery mode approximately every 90 minutes within our daily rhythm when repair of cells and replenishment of energy resources occur. It occurs on a deeper level through our sleep cycles. In fact, it even happens on a moment-to-moment basis with every breath inhaled and exhaled. One needs and supports the other, with one flowing into the other. Energy is optimised when we live with our cycles and rhythms, rather than against them. But the nature of our modern lifestyles constantly pulls us in the direction of adrenalised energy. It keeps us locked in that mode. Relaxation no longer comes naturally. In fact, we don't even know what real relaxation feels like anymore. We must consciously retrain it back into our system in a systemised way as if we are learning a brand-new skill. Relaxation needs to become a discipline.

Only then can we become skilled at using adrenalised energy constructively by harnessing and focusing it and consciously breaking out of it when it's no longer appropriate. By understanding our natural energy patterns and honouring the time to rest and recover, we can adjust our lifestyle accordingly.

Jack reflected on what his energy pattern was like on an average day. It made sense to him to tailor his tasks and plan his diary so that he matched his tasks to his daily energy pattern.

The hour just before sunrise was a time when his creativity seemed to flow most strongly. He would use this time to create, journal and self-reflect. It worked for him to get into the office early and tackle his emails before everyone else burst into the office and demanded his attention. A light breakfast and espresso was the energy boost he needed at around 9am just before his meetings began for the day. He knew that by 3:30pm his energy would start to dip, so he planned his least demanding meetings and tasks for this part of the day, and the activities that demanded the least focused attention. Although Jack's lifestyle was demanding, relaxation came easily for him when he was in an environment that supported it.

It was as if he had a natural pliability in his energy states, an ability to experience both ends of the energy spectrum. His challenge was learning to become far more finely tuned to how he was feeling so that he could consciously shift his energy to a mode that was most appropriate in each situation. But this awareness necessitated a slowing down and tuning in to the sensations in his body, for example, the dryness in his mouth and tension in his shoulders when he was adrenalised versus a sense of peace and calm focus when he was relaxed. Part of his energy management strategy was to become more skilled at recovery loops, which is the art of consciously activating the relaxation response to recharge, rejuvenate and fuel up for the next high-energy cycle. It was imperative that he was conscientious about these recovery loops and that he designed his life in a way that made space for them daily, weekly, monthly and quarterly.

He found that Saturdays worked as a day to slumber, soak up the sun and fit in some exercise, but his challenge was to find a way to integrate shorter recovery loops into each day. Now that he was becoming more cognizant of the subtleties of his energy states and rhythm, Jack noticed the people, environments and situations that supported his energy states and those that drained them. He also became aware of the patterns of thought and behaviour that influenced it. This opened up more choices and possibilities of how he chose to spend his time and what he committed to. Instead of fighting occasional 'low' energy cycles, he used them as opportunities to slow down his pace and consolidate rather than create and start new projects. In his periods of slowing down, Jack started to experience calm moments that he could only describe as a feeling of expansion, clarity, greater perspective and inspiration.

The law of Stillpoint was at play.

Stillpoint is like the eye at the centre of the storm. It is the feeling of freedom and calm from anxiety. It's a feeling that we all crave and strive to achieve and yet is actually always there. Navigating change and the complexities of life is an invitation to anchor to a place inside ourselves, and stretch into the demands of the world from there. Every now and again, we tap into this place through a fleeting moment that arrives quite unexpectedly while walking barefoot on the beach, watching a sunrise or sunset, or listening to the rain. We feel it when we're pulled into a moment. The more we experience Stillpoint, the more we are able to manage times of adversity and change with grace and equanimity. Stillpoint connects us to the source of natural energy or life force energy. The more we tap into it, the more authentic energy can be expressed physically, mentally and emotionally. Experienced martial artists, master creatives and peak sports performers describe this feeling of being 'in flow' or 'in the zone'. We can channel tremendous power, strength and energy by being connected to natural energy.

The concept of Stillpoint resonated with Jack. And he also knew that he hadn't experienced that feeling enough lately. Being in the company of trusted friends, trail running through forest paths and certain music carried Jack to a place of equanimity and stillness that fed his body, mind and heart for a long time. He was aware of the importance of harnessing this principle and wanted to create more opportunities to experience it without making any special effort to manufacture them. In fact, it dawned on him that every moment was an opportunity to experience Stillpoint. All that was required was the ability to be more present in more moments.

Jack was ready to learn about the third law – the law of three channels – which is the expression of authentic energy through mind, body and heart intelligences. There is an innate intelligence that guides and coordinates all our physiological processes and functions without us having to think about it. To support this mechanism, we simply need to take of care of our basic needs and as much as possible live in accordance with natural rhythms. With Jack, we had already done much of this groundwork through working with body awareness and recovery loops. Now we were ready to look at how to optimise his mind intelligence. Focus, concentration, willpower, intellectual capacity, innovation, logical thinking and creativity are all sharpened when we practise the art of attention. Focused attention to everything we are relating to moves us out of knee-jerk reactivity and allows us to be more responsive to ourselves, people and situations. We foster greater resilience when we break out of habitual patterns of thinking and behaviours that trigger reactivity and toxic adrenalised energy.

A natural consequence of a healthy body and clear, focused mind is heart intelligence. We are far more likely to tap into our natural, open-hearted state once we have supported our body's basic needs and are not behaving in a fear-based reactive way. The qualities of heart intelligence are compassion, gratitude, creativity, capacity to feel and connect with ourselves and others without judgement. To harness the law of three channels means to be consciously in attendance to them each day. Tending to one channel will influence all the others. It is all one interconnected system.

Jack noticed that sometimes when he was feeling anxious and stressed, it helped to get out of the office and take a walk. There were other times when all he needed was some silence and five minutes of deep breathing. Without knowing it, he was applying Newton's law, the 4th law of energy.

Every thought, feeling and emotion that we experience has its own energy pattern. The way that we move, think, feel and breathe has an effect on how we experience energy. When we understand this, we can use this law to transform stress energy or adrenalised energy into something useful. For example, we can transform scattered mental energy or anxiety into authentic energy through physical exercise, or we can transform emotional energy into creative energy through writing or painting. Another example is how we can use positive self-talk (mental energy) to boost physical energy. When we express our feelings through laughing, crying, dancing or talking, we are freeing stuck emotional energy in a physical way. Children do this naturally. Like heat can transform solid water to vapour, the breath is a simple and effective way to transform adrenalised energy to authentic energy through the three channels. A healthy energy system requires that there is a constant flow of energy through the body, mind and heart.

Now Jack's challenge was to craft a lifestyle that worked in harmony with his unique psychobiological pattern, the law of unique you. While there are universal principles that govern energy, we all have unique needs and life circumstances. For example, an extrovert might feel energised by being in a crowd, while an introvert would find being in a crowd exhausting. We have the ability to design a lifestyle and create an environment that supports and honours our individual needs. This requires introspection, awareness and experimentation!

To understand what this meant for Jack, we looked for clues in an ancient science of healing called Ayurveda. It is a science and a way of life that originated in India more than 5000 years ago, but that still has relevance today. Like many other ancient systems, Ayurveda provides a framework of understanding to support our individualised body–mind patterns and honours our cyclical natural rhythms. It is a guidance system for working with our bodies as a sophisticated and interconnected mind–body mechanism.

Each person, as part of nature, has a unique energetic pattern based on our genes, upbringing, environment, diet, belief systems, personality, unique talents and our souls' purpose. Homeostasis or balance is maintained by our system constantly fine-tuning our adaptation to the internal and external environment according to this specific morphological, physiological and psychological blueprint. We are a unique creation of physical appearance, metabolism, personality and preferences, and as such, we all have differing needs and varying ways in which we can support our natural energy. There isn't a 'one size fits all' approach. While systems are helpful to cultivate deeper awareness, it would be naive to assume that Ayurveda, or any other system, can deliver all the answers we want.

In Jack's case, however, it does provide some valuable clues. Ayurveda would classify Jack is a Pitta (Fire) type, in line with his forward-charging spirit, intensity and passion for life. This also correlated to his fast metabolism. He didn't tolerate skipping meals well and would easily get irritable as his glucose levels dipped. To keep his 'fire' in check, he needed to maintain constant and adequate hydration. Hot spicy food, alcohol and caffeine fuelled this fire and manifested as heartburn and headaches. Meals were either shoveled down on the go or enjoyed at a slighter slower pace in restaurants where the focus was conversation. This way of eating confused his 'gut intelligence' even more.

Once he cultivated a clearer understanding of his body type, he was able to adjust his lifestyle in accordance with it. For Jack, his morning routine was adjusted to begin the day with a calm focus. He made the effort to hydrate more throughout the day. In terms of exercise, swimming and a slow form of yoga was the perfect combination for Jack. The swimming took care of his cardiovascular exercise while balancing his excessive 'fire' energy at the same time. A slow form of yoga was ideal to help him to be grounded, connect with his body, breathe deeply and detoxify. Being highly creative and intelligent meant that Jack used his mind in a particular way that was quicker than most. Sometimes this worked for him and at other times it meant that he was distracted, impatient and missed out on meaningful moments. Mindful living became the key to harnessing his logic and magic and cultivating true resilience.

Now he needed to apply the 6th law, the law of flow.

Nature accepts challenges as a stimulus for growth through a process of adaptation and resilience. Likewise, when we can flow with the challenges and difficulties we face without recoiling or building up emotional defences and walls, we tap into our innermost energy resources that can stimulate even greater growth and development.

As I walked through the streets with Jack, it was very clear that his greatest source of authentic energy came from his heart and his connection with the people who live and work in the precinct. Through this mixed-use development, he had created a sense of belonging for himself and for so many people. The young entrepreneurs that he mentored, the local and foreign artists and the visitors from the suburbs constantly fed his heart intelligence. As a leader, taking responsibility for maintaining this connection would ensure that the 7th law naturally expressed itself.

The 7th law, or law of overflow, relates to the phenomenon of entrainment that we see reflected in nature when birds fly together in unison or when women who live in close proximity start to synchronise their menstrual cycle. This law of physics states that when two objects of like vibration are in close proximity, the object of lesser or weaker vibration will begin to match the object of stronger vibration. Thus, if each person takes responsibility for living with authentic energy, this energy state overflows and positively influences the environment and others without effort. The more people that interact on this level, the greater the influence this authentic energy becomes. This is how each person has the capacity to change and grow teams, organisations, family and societal systems.

Jack began to put the energy laws into action. By tuning into his body, he became more aware of its soft whispers and less than subtle screams. Tweaking and adjusting his lifestyle according to his energy cycle reaped great short-term benefits but will also pay great dividends as the pace of his life becomes even more demanding.

The seven laws of authentic energy

Our relationship with our body, our vehicle of energy, is like a good relationship or friendship. We get to know each other over time. And over the years, this relationship matures and deepens. We start making choices that are supportive of its growth and we respect its needs. The understanding of our body occurs through trial and error, and sometimes by making the 'wrong choices'. It's all part of the process, a process that begins with an awareness and that deepens when we can apply the natural laws that govern energy.

1. *Law of rhythms:* Energy moves in rhythms and cycles. In nature, there is a constant oscillation of a high energy state and a relaxation state. In our neurobiological system, we experience this rhythm as adrenalised energy governed by the sympathetic nervous system and the relaxation/rest mode governed by the parasympathetic nervous system. Our survival is dependent on the balance of both. Authentic energy is experienced when we work with the law of rhythms rather than against it. This means being able to constructively use adrenalised energy and knowing when and how to rest and recover through recovery loops.

2. *Law of Stillpoint:* Stillpoint is a moment in time when the noise of everyday life is filtered out and a state of deep peace, joy and wellbeing-centred aliveness or authentic energy is felt. Movement, growth and expansion is dependent on the law of rhythms but also on the anchoring to the feeling of stillness. We experience this in nature, in a calm environment or when we are pulled into a present-moment experience. Through Stillpoint we access the source of authentic energy. We feel peaceful, joyful, compassionate, calm, inspired and tuned into our gut feelings. In order to master our energy system, we have to consciously create, choose and prioritise more Stillpoint experiences.

3. *Law of three channels*: Source energy is expressed through three channels: the body, mind and heart. These dimensions

of energy are all inter-connected and all need to be attended to and supported at any given time, some more than others.
4. *Newton's law:* Energy cannot be created nor destroyed, but changes from one form to another. Energy is never constant. It's always moving and changing forms. When energy becomes stagnant, stuck or scattered, we experience it as fatigue, illness, frustration or anxiety. We can support better flow when we develop the skill of harnessing our energy and directing it in various ways using body, mind and heart intelligences. For example, we can transform mental energy into physical energy or physical energy into emotional energy.
5. *Law of unique you:* No one person is the same. We are all a unique expression of energy based on our genetics, culture, environment, personality and instinctive nature. Thus we each require slightly different ways and methods to support and express our energy. Energy mastery requires that we develop enough self-awareness to design an energy strategy that is unique to you.
6. *Law of flow:* Nature does not resist adversity but faces it, adapts to it and then flourishes. Authentic energy is experienced when we can allow adversity to deepen our capacity to feel and connect with ourselves and others, rather than recoiling in fear, hardening up and building defensive strategies. This merely prevents natural energy from flowing.
7. *Law of overflow:* When we live with more authentic energy, we become a source of energy ourselves. It 'overflows' from us and without trying, positively influencing everything and everyone around us.

Plot yourself on the energy zone map on page 4. What zone are you in at the moment? How long have you been here? What does your energy rhythm look like? What part of the day do you feel most energised? When do you feel most tired? Now think about your weekly energy rhythm. Do you have time in the month when you are most energised? Is your energy pattern seasonal? What is your energy signature? What do you believe influences it? What and who gives you energy? Who and what drains your energy? What brings you a sense of stillness and peace? How often do you give time to the experiences that support this feeling? What source of energy do you believe requires the most attention right now? Body, mind, heart?

> Energy Formula
> *Seven laws of authentic energy + awareness = authentic energy*

Body Intelligence

CHAPTER 2

The intelligent pulse of life (IPOL)

*Every single cell in the body is working tirelessly
to keep the system functioning optimally
according to the perfect blueprint of health
with which we were born.*

SERENA'S STORY: IPOL AT WORK
Name: Serena du Toit
Age: 38
Character traits: Determination and empathy, inability to say 'no'
Life-changing experiences: Premiere of first ballet performance, near-death experience after gastric haemorrhage
Stress catalysts in last two years: Work pressure and piloting of new trauma project through the Emergency and Medical Services
Stress indicators: Headaches, anxiety and insomnia
Presentation on energy zone map: Burnout zone

Her name is Serena, which means one who is composed, peaceful and cheerful. She knows that she felt this way once. Long ago. But she can't remember when. She has spent the last decade stamping out blazes across the city, rescuing families and saving homes. She's seen fires in townships, turning shacks to ash in minutes. She's watched buildings burn and people burn. She's witnessed the anguish on the faces of those who have lost their homes and terror on the faces of little children who have lost everything they knew.

Now the fire is inside her, out of control and devastating. There's not much left to burn.

She's sitting on the porch, the African sun warm on her neck. The air is swaying to its own silent rhythm. Bruised jacaranda flowers scattered on the grass are evidence of a wild night of thunderstorms. She doesn't notice. Once again, she's been wide eyed all night with the creatures of the dark and electrified air, flirting with the idea of ending it all. The shock of the thought jolts her back to her body, her awareness shifting between the waves of nausea and the vice grip around her skull. She hasn't slept in days. The shadows under her eyes match the green within them. Her body has never let her down. Until now. Her mind has always been a source of strength. Until now.

She wonders how it ended up like this and her mind flashes back to how it began, the day that she swapped her ballet shoes for safety boots. Now the only pirouettes are the thoughts in her mind, spinning out of control. The face of her ballet teacher flashes through the spin and her headache intensifies. She remembers her fierce determination to expand and grow past the limits of her elfin physique. She remembers the feeling of freedom she felt when she was on stage, graceful arms stretched into air, eyes bright with hope and fairy-dust freckles sprinkled across her cheeks. However, she realised even then that being a ballerina was not what was written in her stars. The shattering of that dream revealed her innate knowing that she wanted to make a difference in the world. She dreamed of being a doctor, of being in a blue scrub uniform in the trauma unit, of giving back life just before it got lost too soon. The trauma unit is where she would have stayed. That wasn't written in the stars either. Being a firefighter was the next obvious choice. It was another way she knew she could make a difference and perhaps it was even more exhilarating. The adrenaline became addictive.

As the sun stretches across the post storm sky, Serena sighs in bewilderment at the thought of how the demands of the job and life have turned her passion into poison. Two years ago, when she woke up in a hospital bed with a bleeding peptic ulcer, she knew that she needed to slow down. It was just around that time that Gezina, her beloved Labrador, appeared in her life. It was a birthday gift from her husband. Gezina seemed to have been born with a gift of healing and guided her career in a completely new direction. Serena noticed that he naturally gravitated to children who were in pain physically and emotionally. His mere presence seemed to be balm for a broken heart.

It was then that she stepped out of the field and began working in training and fire safety education. Gezina was the perfect partner. She initiated a pilot project involving the use of dogs like Gezina to assist trauma cases involving children. Nothing compared with the moment when the eyes of dog and child locked, the moment of a miraculous healing. That was the moment when her heart softened and she knew without a shadow of a doubt that she was exactly where she needed to be.

With driving out to schools, educating, training, piloting projects, writing reports, taking care of David, her son, managing the household, Serena became the expert juggler. At night, after ensuring that tummies were full, the lullabies were sung and the world had gone to sleep, the textbooks opened up until the early hours. It felt good. Adrenalised energy always does at the beginning. Insidiously, the stress began to accumulate and within a few months, her body began to grumble. She had less energy: she was snapping at David more often and was beginning to feel like a bad mother. And she forgot that she was a wife. The headaches were starting to become a constant companion.

That day, emerging through the searing pain in her head, came the realisation that her health was in a dire place, much more than it was when she was hospitalised. So much energy was depleted in the effort to keep her headaches at bay. They began as a vague threat as soon as she got out of bed and built up to an excruciating crescendo by the end of the day. Pain was a constant companion. Sleep was almost impossible. She ate practically nothing but started gaining weight. She hadn't had a period in months. She had hoped she was pregnant but knew it was unlikely. Her oestrogen levels were at postmenopausal levels. Her heart thumped against her tiny ribcage as a reminder that her body was in trouble. Anxiety gave way to numbness. But the anxiety was more familiar. Being busy, productive and getting things done made her feel safe ... and worthy. Too many people needed her and if she didn't keep it all together, who would? She heard the water go on in the shower and it dawned on her that she hadn't even started breakfast or packed lunches. There was no time for this pity party. She just needed to get through this week. Just one more exam and then she was on her way to getting her psychology degree. Maybe then things would get better.

When I first met Serena, she smiled cautiously through the discomfort I knew she was in. She was in her blue heavy firefighter's uniform, a little baggy for her small frame. Gezina sat next to her protectively, his deep brown eyes following me curiously. In her hand was a big brown envelope with a cross-sectioned picture of a brain. It offered no clue to the cause of the headaches.

We began with an enquiry into her life. She was in trouble. Despite her body being strong and resilient, she had taken herself to the edge. Her cortisol levels were worryingly high. Cortisol is a hormone secreted by the adrenal glands in response to stress. Levels are usually higher in the morning to boost us into action and wane towards the afternoon. In healthy doses, it provides energy and improves memory but high doses over a long period cause havoc. It suppresses thyroid function, lowers immunity and affects the control of glucose. Prolonged high doses can cause insulin resistance and the accumulation of belly fat from the inhibition of the body to burn fat for energy. This is exactly what Serena was experiencing. Her oestrogen levels were still low and she was borderline diabetic. Chronic inflammation had set into her system, which is a typical response to stress. Her body had kicked into self-preservation mode, hungry for any source of energy. She had been operating on adrenalised energy for so long that the body's ability to retain homeostasis had become overwhelmed. The constant surge of adrenal hormones kept her muscles locked in spasm. She could hardly breathe. The only time she was aware of her breathing was when the anxiety set in and she was gasping for air. Whenever she did eat, it was a banana, maybe a sandwich. Just something to keep going, a means to an end. She liked the fact that hunger was a rare urge. Feelings of being overweight had always been an issue, ever since ballet school.

For a long time, Serena's body had been whispering that something was amiss, but she was pushing too hard to notice. The day she landed up in hospital with the bleeding stomach ulcer was when she acknowledged that she needed to take better care of herself. But before long, it was all forgotten and she was back on her horse, studying, working, running the home and being at the beck and call of anyone who needed her. Everyone knew that they could always depend on Serena and that she would never say no. Serena became her own worst enemy and she had almost given up the fight. But not quite.

In our session, she shared how through her work with Gezina and the children, she got to witness the incredible power of nature and that miracles unfolded right in front of her on a daily basis. I reminded her that she is a part of that very same miracle.

Every second of every day and with every single breath that we take, 400 billion bits of information are being processed. Every one of our 100 trillion cells is like its own planet, communicating with all the other cell planets in the galaxy – microcosm of the macrocosm. A million biochemical, enzymatic, immunological and endocrine functions are at work every second. Each system has its own job description, yet is exquisitely coordinated to keep us alive.

What is the intelligence that tells the heart to send white cells racing off to the site of an infection? Is it the same intelligence that makes us yawn when we're tired, and gets the pineal gland to secrete the sleep hormone in response to darkness? Is it the same intelligence that stimulates milk from a mother's breast at the sound of her baby crying? Is it the same intelligence that in one millisecond facilitates the processing of light signals through the retina, sound signals through the perfectly designed ear down the auditory nerve and to the brain, keeps the heart beating, the lungs pumping, the liver detoxifying and the stomach digesting? Could it be the same intelligence that changes the chemical composition of happy tears and sad tears? Could it really be the very same intelligence that gives superhuman powers to a woman to lift a car off her trapped baby? Is it possible that it is the same intelligence that runs through all forms of life and that coordinates signals within all of existence?

I think it is and so I call her IPOL, the intelligent pulse of life, which is the pulse of life within us that is part of the pulse of life around us. IPOL is authentic energy. She expresses herself in the most astonishing ways in the miraculous mind-body machine that is us.

Despite our unnatural ways of living, the toxic air that we breathe and the nutrient-void processed food that we consume, every single cell in the body is working tirelessly to keep the system functioning optimally according to the perfect blueprint of health that we were born with. Most of the time, it does pretty well, even when we don't do much about it. When we're young, healthy and energetic, it's easy to take IPOL for granted. Many of us are not even aware of its existence. As long as we're getting through the tasks of the day, we let the body do its thing. IPOL is generous. It gives us enough time and opportunity to do what needs to be done, respectful of the fact that we are living in a time of thinking, a time where all of life feels like a high-demand situation.

However, there comes a time when IPOL gently nudges us into the awareness of the simple need to maintain this perfect system of health, balance and energy. These nudges show up as the niggling digestive issues like heartburn, bloating and constipation. It shows up on the skin. It tells us that something is amiss when we don't feel as energised and optimistic as we used to. It's IPOL that is speaking to us when we wake up at 3am and can't fall asleep until it's time to wake up. It is nothing but IPOL starting to raise its voice a little louder when the heart thumps hard against the chest. 'Not a heart attack yet,' it shouts, 'but if you don't give me what I need to do my job, I will become one.'

IPOL has a persistent and nagging voice but we have found bizarre ways to shut it up and placate it for a while with anti-inflammatories, anti-spasmodics, anti-hypertensives and anti-biotics. We think we're doing really well when we have our cholesterol checked and unquestioningly fill out the scripts written by well-meaning doctors. We pour ice water over the hot spots. We muffle the voice of IPOL so that we can get on with the business of being busy.

Despite all the neglect, IPOL does its best to maintain and preserve life. However, when the system in which it operates becomes so depleted and toxic that it can't do its job, it turns on the siren, sometimes bringing our whole system to an abrupt halt. In other words, when the body's ability to maintain homeostasis becomes overwhelmed and its compensatory mechanisms occur for prolonged periods, it is at the expense of long-term health.

Serena heard her own siren and that's when she decided to see me. I reminded her that the requirements for IPOL to maintain authentic energy are simple and basic like nature itself. I shared with her that within all the complexities of the human form and experience lies a profound simplicity and that if we simply take care of some fundamentals, IPOL not only supports optimum health but also supports the body to become the vehicle for us to express our highest selves.

She was disturbed by the awareness of how she was disregarding her body's essential needs. We decided just to support her recovery process by focusing on the fundamentals. She made a commitment to make some changes. What would happen to her symptoms if she just focused on these basic pillars? The process proved to be more challenging than she initially anticipated. Some of her lifestyle patterns had become so hardwired and deeply entrenched that breaking them required commitment, conscious awareness and consistency.

Making the effort to eat breakfast was the simple beginning, and IPOL responded by kick-starting her metabolism for the rest of the day. She became more aware of the midday tummy grumbles and succumbed to the need to eat. She ensured that she kept her water bottle close while Gezina panted beside her, reminding her to breathe. By consciously reducing her caffeine intake and creating a winding-down ritual before bed, her sleep quality began to improve and her circadian rhythms got back into sync. One morning, as she was sitting at her desk working on a report, she noticed that something felt strangely different. The realisation dawned that she was headache free, for the first time in months. Within three weeks her headaches lessened in frequency and intensity, and her energy levels began to lift. She was astounded that this was all it took. She was amazed at how her body began to come alive through these simple changes.

Supporting her basic needs was all it took for Serena to recover. Her body proved to be resilient and very responsive to the support it was beginning to get. Now when she feels the familiar tight feeling at the back of her neck and she feels her shoulders creeping up to her ears, she simply stops to listen to the voice of IPOL. She soon began to feel the same energy and enthusiasm for life that she was used to. Through yoga she woke up the old memory of freedom in her body that she used to feel when she was on the ballet stage. Attending to the basic pillars of health provided a new architecture for IPOL to move through. It felt like a cool flame of awareness and her spirit came alive. Serena was back. Composed, peaceful and cheerful.

The basic needs for optimum functioning of IPOL

1. Food that slowly and steadily releases glucose, a basic unit of energy to the cells. Food that is nutrient dense and rich with all the fats, proteins, vitamins, minerals and enzymes needed to

support all the other complex functions of the cells.
2. Oxygen is required by the cells to burn food to provide energy to sustain life.
3. Water is essential for detoxification, cleansing and excretory functions, thermal regulation, maintenance of electrolyte and acid base balance. It also serves as an important transport medium for nutrients.
4. Exercise optimises weight and functioning of all the body's systems. Exercise makes IPOL shine, move and thrive!
5. Sleep of an adequate restorative nature is vital for all the rejuvenative functions of the body to occur.

Needless to say, we all have a unique genetic makeup and individual story. Some of us will require more specific nutritional, medical or even surgical intervention. However, do not underestimate the power of IPOL to restore and regenerate the system. That's what it has been designed for. It just requires us to supply the basics. Now, more than any other time in our history, it is a vital requirement that we prioritise and support the basic pillars of health.

There was a time when these simple needs where just that – simple and obvious. We didn't need to write books about them. Our lives were far more in tune with nature and we honoured the natural rhythms of our bodies. Food was preservative free and the air was clean. We knew how to relax. What used to be obvious isn't obvious anymore.

What language is your IPOL speaking?

Do a body mapping process to better understand what language your IPOL is speaking. Take a large sheet of paper and draw an outline of your body. Using different colours, shade and mark where you are experiencing pain or discomfort. Note where you have had problems in the past. Mark the places where you have had any injuries or operations. What have you become aware of? Has IPOL been trying to tell you something?

Checking in on the basics

Go back to the basic needs above and write down how you believe you are able to support each pillar a little better. Are you ready to commit to putting any of these into action? What support do you require to make these changes?

> Energy Formula
> *Basic needs + IPOL = authentic energy*

CHAPTER 3

Eating for authentic energy

Our relationship with food is often a reflection of our deep and complex relationship with ourselves.

> **LEO'S STORY: THE FOOD THAT LOVES YOU BACK**
> **Name:** Leo Angelis
> **Age:** 32
> **Character traits:** Compassion and aggression
> **Life-changing experiences:** Summiting Kilimanjaro, witnessing a double rainbow perfectly suspended between two cliffs somewhere in the Mediterranean
> **Stress catalysts in last two years:** Quitting a corporate job, legal dispute and court case with previous corporate employer
> **Stress indicators:** Back pain, joint pain and stiffness, abdominal cramps
> **Presentation on energy zone map:** Danger zone

The air is thick with tropical heat; the sun has just started to slip behind the ocean. Sticky juice from a ripe mango seeps through his fingers and down his stubbled chin as he sucks on its flesh. He wiggles his toes deeper into the sand to find a cool spot. The contrast between his skin and the tattooed symbol on his arm has faded from lying in the sun all week. Coconut palms sway in the light breeze. The moment expands, making space for even more bliss. Leo Angelis has never felt more alive.

This is Leo's first trip to India, booked on a whim. It's been a soul-destroying year, consumed by a drawn-out legal battle with his previous employer. India seemed like an obvious choice for a break – exotic and far enough from everything, away from the grip of frustration that had kept him feeling exhausted and ill for almost a year. Now, the sound of the ocean caressing the shore is trance-inducing, washing away all memories of stress.

A beach vendor strolls past, coconuts tied to either end of a pole resting lightly on his shoulders. Aaaah, fresh coconut water, who could resist? After one perfect swipe of a knife and exchange of a coin, the top of the coconut is hacked and the cool water slips down Leo's throat. He's already fantasising about dinner, of freshly caught prawns grilled in butter and Goa's famous Portuguese-inspired peri-peri sauce. From the moment of his arrival in Mumbai, every sense is being challenged and stretched, leaving little room for imagination. His taste buds are on full alert, ready to embrace the next flavour. Tangy tamarind, sweet coconut, heady cardamom and saffron merge through the meals and linger through the day. Mounds of fragrant rice are served with a variety of curries on banana leaves as plates.

With the promise of dinner just a couple of hours away, Leo slowly unfurls himself, dusting the sand off his shorts. He flings his towel over his shoulder and, with a lazy stride, makes his way up the beach and through the gardens up to the bungalow. There's time for a nap before dinner. Leo flops down and sprawls out, his mind drifting to the edge of a dream. Within 15 minutes he is jolted awake with the familiar rumbling just under his belly button. Then, like a firecracker, the pain shoots up under his ribcage. Sparks of hot light fire up a chain reaction of pain across his abdomen and into his chest. His breath ceases. He is on his knees at the edge of the bed, in the space between prayer and pain. He reaches for his cosmetic bag, rummaging through the bottles to find the box of antispasmodics. Leo knows this pain well. It's a stark reminder of his unrequited love affair with food. He was hoping that being on holiday would somehow change things. Today's attack is particularly vicious. Usually, the irritable bowel syndrome plays up as a vague discomfort, a 'barely there' ache that sends his energy through a downwardly spiraling vortex. He spends the rest of the night writhing and dipping into sleep between waves of pain.

He wakes up groggy and exhausted. Maybe a walk along the beach would help. He finds himself on a dusty side road on his way down a path that seems like it could have been a shortcut. He forgets his pain for a while as he is pulled into all the bustling activity of the hippy town and stops at the chai stand, the aromas of fresh ginger and spice blends with the lingering incense. His gaze lands on a sign that reads: 'Dr Ravi Ram, Ayurvedic Physician'.

Leo remembers hearing about Ayurveda from one of his friends who had come to an Ayurvedic detox centre in India the previous year in an attempt to deal with an alcohol dependence. Before long he is sitting in front of Dr Ravi, whose oversized eyes spill over the top of rimless glasses. He answers some questions about his diet, lifestyle and personality, and after a rather long study of Leo's pulse, Dr Ravi announces that he is a typical Kapha (Earth) type. With his easy-going nature, calm and loving disposition, and tendency to gain weight, it is easy for Dr Ravi to make this assessment. However, all the stress and uncertainty of the past year has caused a current Vata (Wind) imbalance as well. This would explain why his digestive system was playing up more than usual. He hands Leo a typed sheet with a Kapha diet, which contains a list of foods that will help restore his body back to health, maintain his weight and sustain his energy levels.

Leo is left feeling even more anxious and confused as his eyes scan the page. He doesn't even recognise some of the items on the list that are supposed to be 'good' for him. Some of the items contradict what has been recommended for his blood type, and recently he has read so much about cutting out all grains and changing to a predominantly fat and protein diet. And with his job that requires so much entertaining, how is he ever going to find a diet that maintains his weight, supports his energy levels and prevents his bowel from screaming at him?

A week after arriving back in Johannesburg, Leo slumped down in the chair of my consulting room heavy with questions. What is the best diet to be on? Should he book a colonoscopy? Should he see a dietician? Why does all the advice he's been given around eating seem so conflicting? Why is he so sensitive to so many foods?

After careful enquiry into Leo's current symptoms, diet, eating habits and family history, we began to establish that even though his body's relationship with food was complex, the solution was simpler than he initially thought. Leo's food choices were shaped by a variety of influences. His culture and upbringing, family genetic makeup, his unique body type and biochemistry, busy lifestyle, unconscious eating habits as well as conscious choices all played a role in what he ate. He grew up in a South African Greek family and as first-generation immigrants many family meals were strongly inspired by the Mediterranean way of cooking. His mother was a passionate and traditional cook who found great pleasure in creating abundant fresh meals and decadent desserts. They always ate together as a family, and dinners were long and leisurely, peppered with much flavour and conversation. Like his mother, his passion and zest for life has always been reflected in his relationship with food. However, through the years Leo noticed that eating certain kinds of bread and dairy products would trigger abdominal spasms, allergic symptoms and nasal congestion. With difficulty, he attempted to avoid both. Both his father and sister had the same experience and he suspected that this was something he had inherited. Once he moved out of his parents' home, Leo's eating habits changed. Even though he enjoyed a substantial breakfast of fruit, eggs and toast, he usually bolted out of the house to make it to his first appointment and ended up skipping the first meal of the day. A cappuccino usually carried him through the first few hours, but by 11am, ravenous and like a hungry lion, he sought out any form of sustenance. An early lunch happened on the run, between meetings or during a meeting, where the focus was far from the food. He looked forward to dinner, as his favourite meal would be prepared by his wife if she found the time and energy. If not, it would be a convenience meal, take away or a dinner at a neighbourhood restaurant. They also both loved trying out new places to eat. Usually, one of the meals of the day would fight back with a groan, grumble or scream, sending Leo into a grey spiral of pain and low energy.

As Leo began to tell his story, he was surprised at how much his eating habits had changed over the years. He realised that some changes were necessary. The first thing that we identified was that he was juggling between food that created a temporary energy peak, and comfort food. During the day, he unconsciously opted for anything that would keep him alert and wired. Sugary and spicy foods and caffeine seemed to stimulate his energy during the day when he needed it. At the end of the day, he would somehow crave food that was comforting and satiating. White breads, pasta, potatoes and meat seemed to fill him up when he was running on empty. When he was particularly tired, burgers seemed like manna from heaven. While eating this way gave him temporary comfort, he was always left feeling sluggish and tired the next day. His sinuses felt full and his mind felt dull.

It seemed as if he was unconsciously using food as a way to 'manage' his energy. The sugar, caffeine and spicy food were being used as 'uppers' while the heavy refined carbohydrates and red meat were functioning as 'downers'. Leo's eating pattern was typical of someone functioning on adrenalised energy.

Ayurveda guides our understanding of how this might occur. The ancient science reminds us that nature, and food as part of nature, hold three subtle qualities of energy:

Rajas: This type of energy can be described as adrenalised energy. *Rajasic* energy is restless – stimulating and providing pleasure in the short term, but its peak sets up the scene for a crash that follows it, thus causing imbalance. Caffeine, sugar, heavy spices and preservatives are examples of food that agitates and creates turbulence in the body and mind.

Tamas: This state can also be described as 'inertia'. It holds the force of heaviness, stickiness and obstruction. Eating food with *tamasic* quality leads to a feeling of sluggishness, dullness and lethargy. *Tamasic* food can also be classified as energy drainers. Over-processed, stale, pre-packed and frozen food and refined carbohydrates like bread, biscuits and pasta fall into this category.

Sattva: Authentic energy or *sattva* is an intelligent source of energy. It is most present in food that is fresh and unprocessed. This energy is drawn from the earth and sun, and thus is abundant in life force. It is light, easy to digest, and brings clarity, perception and balance.

With this understanding of food energies, it made complete sense for Leo to draw on his Mediterranean roots to guide his new way of eating. The Mediterranean diet emphasises eating primarily plant-based foods such as fruits and vegetables as well as whole grains, legumes and nuts, healthy fats and fish, chicken and limited red meat. He realised that for the most part the Mediterranean diet is a *sattvic* diet! If he simply consumed food that was alive with life force and *sattvic* energy, he would be able to access a source of authentic energy.

Through our conversations, Leo also began to see that it was not just *what* he was eating but *how* he was eating that was causing this energy slump. For a long time, he had been racing through his meals in an adrenalised state. Eating on the go had created a habit of gulping water to wash down almost every half-chewed bite. Eating this way did not allow his body to produce sufficient digestive enzymes to break down the food into small enough particles. The digestive juices that were being produced were simply being diluted by all the fluid he was drinking during the meal, reducing their efficacy.

When we are in an adrenalised state, the body's blood supply and energy is directed to the external environment and vital functions and away from the digestive organs. Thus, its functioning is less than optimal and the entire process of digestion and assimilation of nutrients becomes compromised.

In the ideal situation, the digestive dance begins even before the first morsel of food is brought to the lips. The salivary glands are the opening act, squirting their juices into the mouth as the colours and aromas waft up to the olfactory glands, sending signals to them via the brain. This is IPOL in full action. The powerful acidic fire in the stomach is the major and most important part of the act. Any upset to the balance of this process causes the immune system to launch an attack on the food particles that arrive in the intestine. It also places a strain on the liver and pancreas, which are organs responsible for secreting more enzymes into the upper part of the intestine.

The immune system is a powerful defence system directed by IPOL to protect the body from any foreign invader. When it unleashes a ferocious attack anywhere in the body, it creates a devastating inflammation of the tissues around it. The inflammation disrupts the integrity of the bowel wall and the sticky food substances leak insidiously through it, creating a phenomenon known as 'leaky gut'.

In Leo's case, the immune attack in his digestive system was further exacerbated by his genetic predisposition to being wheat intolerant. His body did not produce the enzymes required to digest the modern genetically engineered form of wheat and thus as soon as he ate a wheat product, especially if it was in a refined form, the immune system would attack with even more gusto. The acute spasmodic pain that Leo experienced in India was a battle in a long-standing war. This constant state of inflammation further explained his fatigue, muscle aches and constant sinus congestion.

Leo and I began to design a strategy or way of eating that was fluid, creative, and that would be most supportive for his circumstances and lifestyle. This was the first step in Leo's new relationship with food, his body and his environment. An awareness was sparked that allowed him to make more conscious choices about what he was eating. His love affair with food was rekindled. This time, the love began to flow both ways and the effects were visible.

His mornings begin early, when the sun is still low, with clients often requesting meetings before 8am. So, it works for him to make an on-the-go smoothie packed with seasonal berries, almonds and good-quality protein powder and rice milk, because cow's milk aggravates his sinus congestion.

He is beginning to experiment with all kinds of smoothies made with a variety of greens such as spinach and fennel. Apple and almonds get thrown in too and he is amazed at how long this power breakfast keeps him going. It seems to sustain his energy to the point that he sometimes forgets about coffee. It is no surprise that greens provide such a powerful natural energy boost. The chlorophyll, which gives leaves its green colour, converts the vital energy of the sun and has almost exactly the same chemical composition as haemoglobin in blood!

On slower mornings, Leo makes time for a more leisurely breakfast which comprises a small bowl of fruit followed by an egg on a slice of rye toast and a mug of green tea. He finds that the weather also dictates what he is drawn to eating and on cooler overcast mornings, a sprinkling of grated apple, almonds and honey turns a bowel of warm jungle oats into a colourful culinary concoction.

On days when lunch meetings are not scheduled, Leo is being diligent about packing a substantial lunch box. He has now made it a rule to never eat lunch at his desk or in the car on the run. He is using his mealtimes as opportunities to become more mindful and present. His lunch breaks have now turned into 'meaningful pauses'. He finds that eating in a more relaxed state helps him to become aware of chewing more slowly and that his portions have reduced in size. Now he places far more value on the quality rather than the quantity of food.

Even though he doesn't have a big garden, Leo has started to plant some herbs and even a few vegetables in pots and in a patch in his back garden. Part of his winding-down ritual at the end of his working day is to get into the garden and pick whatever is available for dinner. Suddenly his meals have started to come alive and dinners have become a ritual; a time for connection and conversation. TV dinners are now absolutely forbidden and it has also become a household rule that no phone calls are answered at dinner time.

Leo's new-found love affair with food is contagious. He has inspired his friends and some of his neighbours to begin their own little urban gardens and growing and sharing their own homegrown organic produce has become all the rage!

Since Leo has rekindled his relationship with food, all the digestive symptoms that he had been experiencing for such a long time have practically disappeared and his energy levels have improved considerably. By becoming more mindful and aware, Leo has made the food choices that support him the most. He doesn't always get it right, but now he is far more conscious of how certain foods affect his body and energy levels and is still in the process of refining his choices. In the process, a whole new world has opened up to him. He is learning about all kinds of food choices that he never knew about. Watching how things grow in his garden has deepened his fascination with the perfection of nature.

The business lunches and functions and travelling are still challenging, however, but his new passion has led him to a few food-conscious catering companies and some gentle nudging of his clients to use their services. Just by making this shift in his own life, Leo has created a ripple effect within and around his circle.

Building a good relationship with food

Our relationship with food is often a reflection of our deep and complex relationship with ourselves. As one of our basic human needs, food is a source of nourishment. Like Leo, we can also expand it beyond a basic need to an art form, and a form of creative expression. Sometimes, we use food as a way to punish and deprive ourselves of pleasure, taste and even basic food groups! It often becomes a source of stress. Our relationship with food can easily become contaminated with guilt, self-loathing and shame. So as much as it is a source of nourishment, it can also trigger internal battles, inflammation and ill health. It never ceases to amaze me how many of my patients recover from illness simply by making changes in their food choices and healing their relationship with it. Time and time again, it has been shown that diets that offer miracle weight-loss cures are ineffective and sometimes even dangerous, setting up a vicious cycle of weight loss and then rebound weight gain. In the process disease is driven deeper into the cells. While diets might be short-term solutions to weight loss, they do little to inspire a lasting long-term relationship with the food that truly 'loves you back'.

Eating for energy

What to eat
The Mediterranean way of eating is a good basis from which to begin experimenting with what is best for your body and lifestyle. This means an abundance of fresh vegetables, fruit, lentils, whole grains (bulgur wheat, millet, spelt, brown rice, quinoa), fish, healthy fats (from olive oil, coconut oil, avocados, nuts and fish) and limited red meat and, depending on your constitution, limited organic dairy. Take inspiration from India and incorporate spices like cumin, coriander, cardamom and cinnamon in your meals. Go further east too and try Asian greens like bok choy, fermented soya products like tofu, and exotic mushrooms. Ensure that you incorporate enough items that will support a healthy gut microbiome (bacteria) such as yoghurt with live cultures, sauerkraut and kefir.

Move towards food that is *sattvic* or foods that contain a high concentration of life force. Greens, sprouts and unprocessed food are the most naturally energising.

Avoid using substances that fuel adrenalised energy, spike insulin and cause havoc in endocrine levels like sugar and caffeine.

Limit food that is heavy, difficult to digest and laden with refined carbohydrates, unhealthy fats and processed meats, which all place a strain on the digestive system and cause inflammation.

Become a 'locavore'. A locavore is one who chooses to eat locally produced food as much as possible. Besides supporting the local economy and environment, evidence shows that locally grown produce has a higher nutritional value than produce transported over long distances. A great deal of nutritional value of food is lost in the production, processing and transport of food. Moreover, it seems that the body is more able to assimilate nutrients from food grown closest to your living environment.

Eat seasonally. Our body's needs change according to the seasons and nature's perfect design ensures that these needs are fulfilled when we choose to live in sync with it. Citrus fruit packed with vitamin C is abundant in winter when we are most susceptible to colds. Warm comforting foods like pumpkin and butternut that can be stored for a long time are harvested in the colder months. Juicy refreshing watermelon is heavenly in summer when the sun is beating down.

Eat organic products that haven't been genetically modified (GM-free) as much as possible. The body has an incredibly robust and resilient self-detox mechanism. However, a lifetime of toxic onslaught from food that has been genetically engineered, stabilised and preserved eventually overwhelms this built-in system, and diseases slowly and insidiously get driven deeper into the cells.

How much?

The well-documented Okinawa Centenary study that looked at the factors that were responsible for this group of Japanese people who have shown the highest life expectancy in the world. Their diet seems to be a major factor. Interestingly, it is very similar to the Mediterranean diet, with the inclusion of more fermented soya products. Even more interesting is the Okinawan practice of Hara Hachi Bu or eating only until you are 80% full.

Ayurveda would concur. Eating this way would create more balance between what is consumed and the body's ability to digest it, alleviating the symptoms of bloating and heartburn. We should draw inspiration from the French who tend to draw their meals out with good conversation and as a result end up eating less and staying slim! This makes sense if one considers that it takes 20 minutes for the stretch receptors in the stomach to send the signal to the brain that it's full.

When?
The potency of our digestive juices, like all our physiological responses, are in a constant state of flux and in tune with the rhythm of nature. Once again Ayurvedic wisdom brings to our attention that our digestive rhythm is circadian in its nature, meaning that it follows the sun. When the sun is at its zenith, our digestive strength is at its peak. Having lunch as the main meal with a smaller light dinner is most conducive to good health and digestion. Granted, this is often difficult to adhere to with our modern lifestyles; however, it is helpful to keep this in mind.

How?
Slowing down and practising mindfulness during meals allows us to chew our food better, promoting better secretion of digestive enzymes. Then there is also less need to gulp down copious amounts of liquid with meals. In addition, the tongue is given an opportunity to capture all the wonderful flavours and textures of the meal. When food is interesting and bursting with flavour, we tend to naturally slow down our eating as a way to extract as much pleasure from each bite as possible.

The environment
Both our internal and external environment are equally important if we want to extract the maximum nutritional and energetic value from food. Eating on the run, when adrenalised, angry or anxious, locks down the digestive system. It is helpful to take a moment to calm and centre before eating.

Based on the science of quantum physics, even cooking a meal when in a negative mind space can influence the energetic vibration of the meal and thus have an impact on the people who are sharing it. The external environment can also greatly impact our relationship with food. I love the practice of blessing food as it arrives. Gratitude for the meal, the earth that provided it and the people who prepared it can completely change how the meal is enjoyed.

Mindful eating can turn a meal from being a means to an end to a sacred time to connect and awaken your senses whether you are alone with your partner, with family or a group of friends. Keep a food journal for one week. Make note of the food choices you made and how they have influenced your energy levels and state of mind. Use this and the energy formula below as a basis to make more conscious choices that best support your authentic energy.

> Energy Formula
> *Seasonal* + sattvic + *local* + *mindful* = *authentic energy*

CHAPTER 4

Healthy hydration

Sometimes even more intimate than our relationship to food is our relationship with what we drink.

> **TENJI'S STORY: LIQUID ENERGY**
> **Name:** Tenji Radebe
> **Age:** 36
> **Character traits:** Focus and determination, extreme judgement of herself and others
> **Life-changing experiences:** Moving to Johannesburg
> **Stress catalysts in last two years:** Death of mother and grandmother
> **Stress indicators:** Insomnia, road rage
> **Presentation on energy zone map:** Danger zone

The conference call to London is scheduled to start in 15 minutes. Traffic is at a standstill. The morning business report is not helping matters. The rand has nosedived, sending the market into a spin. She texts her director. At this rate, there is no way she's going to get to work on time, but missing this meeting is not an option. With that thought, Tenji Radebe swerves into the yellow lane and whizzes past the stationary cars to the next traffic light. She manages to weave her convertible BMW back into the mainstream flow. She's making her way to the bank, the organisation that she's been loyal to for the last 10 years. It's no secret that she's been earmarked for directorship.

Both her hands tightly clutch the leather-bound steering wheel as her foot bears down on the accelerator. Now, she's looking for her favourite John Mayer track to play through her Bluetooth. A white minibus taxi stops suddenly in front of her to pick up a passenger. She rams down on her brakes, rolls down the window and shouts vulgar obscenities at the driver. The taxi driver is oblivious. Her jaw clenches and a ripple of tension moves into the muscle under her left shoulder blade. She swerves sharply into the office parking bay and walks into the boardroom with a purposeful stride, looking calm, groomed and focused, just in time for the meeting. Just in time to grab her third cup of coffee.

Meanwhile, on the inside, her body temperature is rising. She can feel the quickening heartbeat in her belly and a wave of nausea rising into her chest. She takes a breath but it fails to reach her lungs. She's got it all under control. Her day has begun. She moves from one meeting to the next, clutching her coffee mug. Coffee gives her the edge. It has always been her magical energy elixir and source of solace. Not today. The one side of her face is going numb and she recognises the appearance of an old and unwelcomed visitor. Anxiety is back. And it's knocking loudly.

By 6pm that evening, Tenji is the one knocking on the door of her best friend's house on an eco estate. By this time, she's on the verge of a full-blown panic attack. Busi was there the last time this happened. She is like a big sister and took on the role even more seriously after Tenji's mother died. Busi has always been there, as a friend, mentor and wise sounding board. Busi sees a reflection of her younger self when she looks at Tenji – dynamic, fierce and determined to prove herself in a world of men. She also knows the price she once paid for working at that pace. Nothing else seemed to matter at the time. She was as single minded as Tenji is now, which is why the alarm bells ring so loudly as Tenji walks in the door. Her eyes are startled, her hands are trembling and she is almost gasping for breath. Busi switches the kettle on, makes Tenji comfortable on her favourite couch and gently guides her into some deep-breathing exercises that she was taught at a retreat she attended a few years ago.

It was Busi who made Tenji's appointment with me. As I introduced myself, I sensed both skepticism and vulnerability behind that poised demeanour. What she felt the night of her first panic attack was so terrifying that she sensed she had no choice but seek help. She knew that if she continued in the same vein, she would end up in hospital and probably in the psychiatric ward. To her, that would be the ultimate failure.

Tenji sat upright at the edge of her seat, listing some generic symptoms. I reminded her that she was not in an interview. She covered a nervous giggle and half relaxed back into the chair. I noticed that her tongue was dry and pale against her mocha skin. Her perfectly manicured nails drew my attention to her delicate and trembling hands. Her body was communicating far more than her words were.

Tenji grew up in a traditional Sotho family and spent her childhood on the outskirts of a small town in the North West province of South Africa. Her mother worked as a domestic worker in Johannesburg. She doesn't remember her father. He died when she was just three years old. She grew up at the feet of her beloved grandmother, who passed away just a few months before. At this point of the story, she pauses and dabs the corner of her eye before the moisture has time to build up into a tear.

Education was always a priority to her, and when she was accepted and received funding to study for a business degree at Wits University, it didn't really surprise those close to her. From a very early age, she always felt like an outsider, she admits. She was never really interested in the frivolous and trivial pursuits of the other children and books always held a far greater appeal. After graduation, Tenji's career took an exponential path. Her natural intelligence, diligent work ethic and social skills were a winning combination. She was headhunted by agencies locally and abroad. The world belonged to her. She had been in a few relationships but found it difficult to sustain any of them. Men were just not a priority. And they all seemed threatened by her anyway. She gave her career everything she had. Her days at the office ended when most others were winding down with their families.

After her grandmother's death, Tenji began spending even more time at work, but not just because of the workload. She's found that, lately, she is taking longer to finish tasks and her thinking has become a little clouded. She also hasn't been sleeping well. Sleep has never been something she's struggled with. Her mid-cycle waking was triggered by her 'to do' list and her bedroom ceiling became the screen for the movie in her mind. Morning bird song was her lullaby for a deep sleep and even the gentle tone that she set on the alarm on her phone felt like a tune of torture.

She only felt semi-alive after her first cup of coffee. The second one got her out the front door. In the mornings, time and hunger were both equally and sufficiently absent for breakfast to be a vague consideration. It was the creamy cappuccino from the cafeteria at work that really did the trick to power her up for the morning. The milk seemed to keep hunger at bay, the sugar spiked her energy levels for a short while and the caffeine did wonders for creative and logical thinking.

'Coffee is my wake-me-up in the morning, my carry-me through the day and my pick-me-up in the afternoon,' she said unapologetically. The fact that she carried a packed lunch was testament to her good intentions to actually eat at midday, but most days it accompanied her back home, untouched. At the end of her long day, and about eight cups of coffee later, Tenji felt wired and exhausted at the same time. She was running on pure adrenalised energy. Her mind held all the information of the day and extracted pieces from it to weave a plan for the next day. She longed for the moment when she turned the key of the front door, kicked off her heels and opened a bottle of her favourite Shiraz. Dinner went from the freezer, into the microwave and down between sips of wine.

When Tenji first came to see me, it was obvious that she was a full blown addict. Caffeine was her drug. So was adrenaline.

Her lifestyle and habits had thrown her into the spiral of a severe sympathetic overdrive and she didn't know how to find her way out. No wonder she was experiencing anxiety. Like Serena, Tenji's foundation of health was crumbling underneath her and she needed support to rebuild it.

It was clear from the very outset that Tenji needed to start the processes of rebuilding her health by doing a gentle detox. Her Pitta (Fire) energy was way out of balance. The rigidity in her body language revealed that her muscle memory had become locked in a long-term stress response. The furrow between her eyebrows told me that her liver was taking strain and the ever-so-slight puffiness under her eyes hinted at the possibility of a compromised kidney function.

Step one was to remove the offending substances. We worked out that between all the coffee, tea and energy drinks, she was consuming at least 800 mg of caffeine and 20 teaspoons of sugar in just one day!

Caffeine content of beverages per cup
Brewed coffee/percolated coffee: 80–130 mg
Instant coffee: 30–170 mg
Single espresso: 75 mg
Ceylon black tea: 58 mg
Chinese Oolong tea: 37 mg
Indian green tea: 38 mg
Coca-Cola: 34 mg
Red Bull: 80 mg

By evening, her body ached and her head pounded. She would give anything to have a full night of restorative sleep. While the coffee may have carried her through the day, it interfered with her sleep quality at night. Caffeine lingers in the body for four to eight hours and with all the caffeine still in her system, it was impossible to switch off at night. That's where the wine came in. Shiraz became her 'get to sleep' ally at the end of her day. And she was needing more and more of it. But by 3am she was wide awake again and only dipped into sleep when it was almost time to get out of bed. Again, coffee was the only thing that came to her rescue. Like many thousands of people across the world, Tenji was addicted to caffeine, the most widely used drug in the world. Coffee is the most popular way for people to get their fix; however, it is also present in tea, colas, green tea, energy drinks, chocolate and some medication.

One only has to visit the Mediterranean to see that coffee drinking is part of a lifestyle and culture. It is enjoyed there in a way that is quite different from the way it is beginning to be used as a way to cope with the demands of life. Caffeine intake in times of stress adds to the duration and magnitude of the stress response. In other words, drinking coffee when already in a stress response puts even more strain on the adrenal glands to produce more adrenaline and cortisol, accelerating the path to burnout. In the short term, caffeine also has the effect of stimulating the release of gastric juices which is why excessive coffee intake can lead to nausea and exacerbate heartburn. Through its effects on adrenaline, the heart muscle is stimulated, raising the blood pressure. Palpitations are not uncommon with excessive usage. However, when it is enjoyed more mindfully and appropriately, caffeine can be the wonderful gift that nature intended it to be.

Tenji relaxed when I said this and we devised a plan for her to still enjoy coffee in a way that was beneficial rather than having a detrimental effect.

The best time to enjoy the first cup of coffee is between 9:30am and 11:30am when the cortisol levels naturally begin to dip. Assuming our natural sleep cycle is intact, the adrenal glands produce a surge of cortisol first thing in the morning. This is the body's natural 'wake me up'. Drinking coffee when the body is already releasing cortisol actually dampens the caffeine's effect, thereby creating a tolerance.

In the next couple of weeks, after the first consultation, Tenji began her detox programme and became far more conscious of her 'drinking' habits. We changed her 'first thing in the morning pick me up' to a cup of hot water with fresh ginger, which helped the body to clear out the toxins that had accumulated during the night. Like Leo, she found that the smoothie idea was a practical breakfast idea. She also found that by the time she got to work, she wasn't craving coffee at all. Her glucose levels were beginning to stabilise from breakfast. At around 10am, she was ready for a cappuccino and enjoyed it as part of a break. She replaced her coffee cup on her desk coaster for her water bottle with a built-in filter and sometimes even put a sprig of rosemary in it to liven up the flavour. If she was feeling her energy wane, and felt the coffee craving coming on, she tried out green tea which she found gave her an invigorating boost. Over the next few days, she became more and more intrigued by the world of herbal teas and experimented with every variety from local Rooibos, Chinese green tea, Argentinian mate and all kinds of infusions. It was as if a whole new universe had opened up to her.

It was imperative that we restored Tenji's natural sleep cycle as part of her pillar of health, and also to break her out of the cycle she was in. Therefore, I discouraged her from consuming caffeine after 2pm. This posed a real challenge as 3:30pm to 5pm was a very vulnerable time when her energy levels really took a dive, despite eating lunch. Most days, she succumbed to her craving with a strong cup of tea with a side of her favourite shortbread biscuits. Herbal tea didn't quite do the trick and the biscuits didn't seem to complement it. We discovered that the afternoon energy slump was more as a result of the dip in glucose than a caffeine craving. An afternoon banana-and-almond smoothie seemed to be the perfect afternoon 'pick me up' and sometimes if she was out of the office, she even tried to get herself a wheatgrass shot.

We decided that it would be best for Tenji to eliminate all forms of alcohol until all her body's natural rhythms had been restored. Chamomile tea was her new 'calm me down'. She still enjoys an occasional glass of red wine, but now it is enjoyed for all its benefits and has become a completely sensory experience.

After about two days of experiencing some symptoms of nausea and headaches, Tenji was amazed at how quickly her energy levels began to lift. She no longer felt anxious, she was able to concentrate and her sleep quality improved dramatically. She woke up naturally without an alarm, feeling refreshed and rested and looked forward to her ginger and lemon infusion. What initially felt like a detox became a way of life.

From our very first moments on earth, our mother's milk is

our initial experience of nourishment; warm, sweet, comforting and nurturing. It's no wonder that as adults we hanker after that same feeling, triggered by ancient memories of long-lost infancy. Sometimes even more intimate than our relationship to food is our relationship to what we drink.

Hydration for authentic energy

IPOL has a system of maintaining a certain level of hydration in our body, extracting water through our fluid and food intake and eliminating it not only through the urinary and digestive system but also through the lungs and skin. IPOL manages to support a perfect homeostasis. When we drink pure water, it is recognised as such and it's absorbed into the blood stream easily. Drinking water assists the kidneys to flush out toxins through the urinary system and supports rather than strains an already overwhelmed excretory system. Plain water is not the only source of hydration, however. We get our fluid intake from everything that we drink (and eat). The problem is that the body has to process everything that comes with the beverage, and therein lies the problem. Even beverages that are marketed as 'healthy' with the use of words like 'vitamin', 'organic', 'pure' and 'light' are laced with hidden sugars, flavourants, colourants and preservatives that all draw on the body's natural energy resources.

Fruit juice might feel like a healthy choice but can cause glucose levels to spike and play havoc with insulin levels. Vegetable juices are less offensive to the glucose–insulin balance. While juices, especially freshly extracted green juices, are brilliant alkanisers and sources of energy and hydration, we can lose out on the natural fibre that is present in whole food. How much water does the body actually require to maintain health and a naturally high energy level? Is it really two litres a day? In fact, the amount depends on body weight, body type, metabolic rate, weather and level of physical activity. For an average person, on an average day, our fluid requirement can be measured according to body weight, in other words, 20 ml/kg/day. So if you weigh 65 kg, your optimal fluid intake would be: 65 x 20 ml = 1300 ml/day

Hydration guide

Water: Drink hot water with fresh ginger, a slice of lemon and some honey first thing in morning. Consume 20 ml/kg/day room temperature or cool water between meals and have small sips during meals.

Coffee: Choose a premium coffee brand, preferably organic and well made. Limit to two cups a day. Avoid coffee after lunch.

Tea: Limit black tea consumption to 1–2 cups/day. Keep daily caffeine intake under 200 mg/day. Avoid black tea after 4pm and be aware of what you consume along with black tea (milk/sugar/biscuits).

Herbal teas: Avoid green tea in the evening especially if you are sensitive to the effects of caffeine. Drink plenty of Rooibos and other herbal teas as they are naturally caffeine free. Drink calming chamomile tea in the evenings.

Wheatgrass juice: A shot daily for 3 weeks with a break of 2 weeks in between.

Vegetable juice: Experiment with different combinations, such as beetroot, carrot, celery, cucumber, spinach, etc. Drink as soon as it's made before it gets oxidized. Most importantly, drink it slowly.

Fruit juice: Drink fruit juices in moderation because of their high fructose levels.

Smoothies: They are a good option as a quick and nutritious meal replacement. Add a good-quality protein powder for an extra boost. Use an abundance of berries and get creative with combinations and flavours.

Energy Formula
Limited caffeine + H2O + 'green' juices + herbal tea
= authentic energy

CHAPTER 5

Sleep and rest

Brain processing and memory consolidation happen as we slumber, enhancing creativity and strengthening neural connections.

> **LEILA'S STORY: NAPS AND DREAMS**
> **Name:** Leila Singh
> **Age:** 23
> **Character traits:** Compassion and stubbornness
> **Life-changing experiences:** Illness and death of grandfather
> **Stress catalysts in the last two years:** Final medical school exams
> **Stress indicators:** Eczema, depression
> **Presentation on energy zone map:** Burnout zone

It's a Sunday morning in late March. The light is changing and the leaves are just starting to turn red and dry on the trees. As church bells ring in the distance, a young intern walks into the hospital ward, greeting the nurses with an unconvincing smile. It's 8am and Leila is on call in the medical unit at a large public hospital in Johannesburg, a concrete slab perched on a hill overlooking one of the largest manmade forests in the world. The beeper goes off exactly three minutes later. Her day begins. She sprints down the stairs to the admissions ward. Steve, her fellow intern, is already there. The queue is beginning to build up. TB, liver failure, asthma attacks, diabetic comas, pneumonia. By 2pm there are no more beds in the admissions ward or the ward upstairs. The passageway is congested with weary patients sitting on chairs, others on stretchers. She finally manages to insert a drip on a sweet 80-year-old woman with elusive veins. Her glucose levels and imagination have soared to new heights. Her next patient is a young 26-year-old man with yellow eyes and a temperature of 40°C, a filmmaker who's just returned from a shoot in Mozambique. She calls the X-ray department for the third time to do a portable X-ray on the patient with an acute asthma attack and then resorts to wheeling the patient down to the X-ray department herself. It is 12 hours since her shift began and she's already admitted 28 patients.

They are sending some patients to other hospitals and discharging others. She does a final walk around the beds and heads to the doctor's restroom at the back of the ward. The mattress sinks in the middle and the sheets feel like they haven't been washed in weeks. Leila always brings her own sheet and pillow when she's on call, which is at least once a week. It offers her a sense of comfort. She hates sleeping away from home and since starting her internship, her life revolves around these seemingly endless 36-hour shifts. The soles of her feet are burning and her lids close over scratchy eyes. It occurs to her that she has forgotten to order blood for the patient who is going to theatre the next day. She'll do it in the morning. The sound of her beeper jolts her upright in a way that would have made Pavlov proud. The nurse's station is calling. Her 80-year-old patient has died. She needs to be certified. No breathing. Pupils fixed and dilated. No pulse. Form signed. Back to bed. Beep beep. Another patient is vomiting blood. Leila walks over to her bed feeling the futility. Vacant eyes stare back through her. She calls her senior for advice. He says he'll try to come past later. He's busy in the ICU, resuscitating a patient who crashed. She orders some blood for transfusion and goes back to bed.

It's 3:30am. She's exhausted beyond the point of rational thought. She's afraid that if she falls asleep now, she might not be able to wake up in time to see her patients before the ward round at 8am. She succumbs.

It's Monday morning and the nurses are handing over to the next shift. There's a piercing wail coming from the corner of the ward. A man is touching the face of the wife who passed in the dead of night, her vacant eyes closed forever. It's 10:30am on Monday and the weary intern has a 'to do' list that is growing as the ward round progresses. By the time she walks in the door of her apartment at 2pm, Leila is bone-weary. She can't decide what to do first; shower, eat, sleep or cry. She cries.

Tuesday and Wednesday are full working days. On Thursday, the 36-hour shift begins all over again.

Leila's real name is Ela Manga. This is my story.

I can't say that I enjoyed being a medical student. It was intense and demanding on so many levels. The incessant pressure to get to the finishing line and to pass the final exams sat heavily on my shoulders. At that time, I was driven mostly by my own desire for achievement. But I also loved people. I was inspired by their stories and was in awe of the miracle that is the human body. I was never at the top of my class, but I worked hard and consistently. I certainly wasn't one of those students who could cram all night and write exams the next day. I remember trying once before an anatomy exam but I didn't make it past 2am. My body and mind have always required eight hours sleep in order to function optimally.

I was one of the lucky interns who was posted close to home, unlike many of my friends who were sent to work in smaller hospitals in rural areas. I began my internship starry-eyed and excited about my future. My plan was that after internship and community service, I would stay in public service to specialise in obstetrics and gynaecology. Like all young interns that came before me and all the young doctors that have come after me, I had to accept that these crazy shifts were simply part of the deal. By the end of my two-year stint at the hospital, I was exhausted, disillusioned and emotionally burnt out. I became desensitised to the suffering around me. My beeper felt like a tool of torture.

Fortunately, my physical health wasn't too badly affected. Perhaps it was the resilience of youth. Or maybe it was just good genes. However, it was the accumulative lack of sleep that took its toll on my emotional health. When I realised that I had disconnected from the feeling of compassion for my patients, I knew that I wouldn't cope with another five years working at that pace, a choice that so many of my colleagues bravely made. I often wonder if I would have made a different choice for my career had I not been so chronically tired. I wonder how the lives of patients and the doctors who care for them are impacted by working these inconceivably long hours with little sleep.

The importance of sleep

Thirty-six per cent of our lives is spent sleeping, equating to 32 years of an average lifespan. With time becoming such an elusive and valued resource, sleep has become the enemy of modern life. The ability to sleep less and do more has become fashionable and desirable. In the process, we have forgotten that sleep is the most important and fundamental source of authentic energy.

Twenty per cent of the world's population are shift workers and suffer the consequences of sleep deprivation, just as I did. But millions of others are affected by sleep deprivation from jet lag, motherhood and as a result of stress, anxiety and being locked in an adrenalised state. We use addictive stimulants like caffeine, sugar and nicotine to keep us functioning during the day, which prevents us from shutting down at night. Then we turn to alcohol and sleeping pills to sedate us at night, but that does little to improve our sleep quality.

A typical anxiety-related sleep pattern is mid-cycle waking up at 2am to 3am in the morning, fighting with a racing mind and then falling into a deep sleep a couple of hours before it's time to wake up. As in Tenji's case, we seek external aids to get us through the morning and the cycle begins again. Another common pattern is either falling asleep in front of the TV in the lounge or TV room and waking up to go into the bedroom or, even worse, using the noise from the TV as a lullaby in the bedroom itself.

For others, it's a challenge to fall asleep at all. Physical pain, medication and an uncomfortable external environment can all influence how much and how we sleep. Many new mothers with babies are at risk of burnout from prolonged sleep deprivation. While we each have differing sleep requirements, research has shown that people who sleep less than six hours a night are at a higher risk for developing chronic illness. In terms of day-to-day functioning, poor sleep quality can severely impact our natural energy levels causing daytime sleepiness, and poor memory, concentration and judgement. Interestingly, lack of sleep has also been linked to weight gain in that it increases the appetite-stimulating hormone ghrelin and decreases the hormone leptin that is responsible for sending signals to the brain when we're full.

Although there is no consensus as to the real function of sleep, we do know that it is a fundamental pillar of health. During sleep, the body rejuvenates and restores itself. It has been found that certain genes linked to cell regeneration and growth are only turned on when we sleep. Brain processing and memory consolidation also happens as we slumber, enhancing creativity and strengthening neural connections. Yet so much of what happens still remains a mystery to scientists.

What we do know is that there is a perfect synchronisation of our sleep cycle with the movement of the sun. Another example of IPOL at work. The pineal gland, a pea-size, cone-shaped gland deep in the brain, acts as our internal timepiece. It contains photoreceptors very sensitive to light signals from the retina and responds to darkness by producing a hormone called melatonin which induces the feeling of sleepiness at night. Light signals are received through the retina from the sun and dampen the secretion of melatonin. This is part of the hormonal cascade that kick-starts our energy in the morning and activates our waking state. Living in an urban setting that is lit up with bright lights, the signal is delayed and sleepiness tends to get triggered later. A fascinating study has recently been done to demonstrate the effect of the lights from televisions, smartphones and tablets that have become the modern-day bed partner. The light from these devices has a direct influence on the pineal gland, which receives a false signal that it is still daytime and therefore can severely impact sleep quality.

During an average eight-hour sleep cycle we go through between four and six cycles of sleep, with each cycle lasting about 90 minutes and having five stages. Every stage has a very distinctive quality, brainwave pattern and purpose. As our head hits the pillow and we begin to make the transition to sleep, the brain waves are small and fast (beta waves). This is close to the brainwaves of the waking state. As the brain waves slow down to theta waves, we slip into stage 1 sleep, which lasts 5–10 minutes. This is followed by stage 2, where we move into light sleep. The body temperature starts dropping and heart rate slows down. In stage 3, the brain produces rapid rhythmic brainwave activity between periods of slow-wave activity. This is when deep restoration work happens in the body. Blood flow to the muscles increases and hormones are activated to stimulate cell growth. We stay here for about 20 minutes before we drop into stage 4, another phase of deep restoration characterised by mostly slow delta waves.

Our dreams occur in stage 5, or REM phase of sleep. This is the most active phase where the brainwaves resemble the waking state and when our muscles periodically go into spasm to prevent us from acting out our dreams. Sleeping pills have been shown to diminish the time spent in REM phase, a vital part of the sleep cycle. Using an alarm clock can also yank us out from the midst of a deep sleep phase and the sleepiness can linger well into the morning. While serious sleep disorders might need more targeted assessment and treatment of the underlying causes, it is helpful to establish a routine that prepares the body for a peaceful and restorative sleep.

Tools for good sleep

Three-step routine for good sleep
Step 1: Establish how much sleep you require. Work this out by establishing how many hours of sleep you need to wake up feeling refreshed without the need for an alarm. This is assuming you have a normal day's activity and have slept well throughout the night. This should be between six and nine hours.

Step 2: Choose a bedtime that will ensure that you are able to wake up naturally without an alarm.

Step 3: Half an hour before your chosen bedtime, begin the wind-down ritual.

Ways to wind down
- Write down your 'to do' list for the next day as well as any thoughts, ideas and inspiration you've had during the day. Enjoy a cup of calming herbal tea such as chamomile. Switch off all electronic devices and televisions.
- Have a warm bath or shower. If you choose a bath, add some Epsom salts to the water. Magnesium eases tense muscles. Alternatively, add some lavender essential oil to the bath or sprinkle it on the shower floor for a soothing aromatherapy shower experience.
- Play some soothing music.
- Mindfulness meditation practice. Do this lying or sitting. Tune into your breath, keep the breath as the focus of your attention. When your mind drifts, bring your focus back to your body and breath. Many of those who experience insomnia become more and more anxious at the prospect of facing yet another night of staring wide-eyed at the ceiling. The anxiety related to not being able to fall asleep feeds the cycle. In other words, 'trying too hard' to fall asleep hinders our ability to slip into sleep. This is why meditation practices assist greatly in breaking the stress cycle and re-establishing natural rhythms.

- Deep slow breathing: Inhale for a count of 4, hold the breath for a count of 7, exhale for a count of 8. See chapter 5 for more details.
- Read some material unrelated to work.

The ideal bedroom environment

Ensure that the temperature in your bedroom is comfortable, that your pillow and mattress are supportive enough. Get breathable cotton linen and bedding that is cool in summer and warm in winter. Banish televisions from your bedroom.

Sleep aids

While it is beyond the scope of this book to go into details around supplementation, sleep aids are commonly prescribed and natural supplements are widely used. However, there is a risk of using supplements indiscriminately.

Valerian: Valerian is a flowering plant whose root has often been used as a sleep aid. It acts as a natural sedative and may be useful for those experiencing insomnia related to anxiety and depression. This has a mild sedative effect and should be used with caution because of possible interactions with other drugs.

Chamomile tea: Drinking chamomile tea has a gentle calming effect and can assist to calm the mind and relax the body.

Lavender essential oil: Add a few drops to your warm evening bath to deepen your relaxation.

Energy nap

The ideal power nap has always been thought to be 20 minutes, but researchers have shown the benefits of a 10-minute recharge nap that immediately improves energy levels, vigour and cognitive performance. Day-time power naps are a great way to boost authentic energy in the middle of the working day and especially in the afternoon when energy levels start to slump.

What stands in the way of sweet slumber

- Drinking caffeine after midday
- Using alcohol as a sedative
- Working on electronic devices or watching television an hour before bed
- Going to bed straight after a meal
- Exercise: Regular daily exercise has a positive impact on sleep quality. However, doing heavy workouts close to bedtime can be quite stimulating and can interfere with the ability to fall asleep.

Energy Formula
Wind down routine + 6–8 hours + power naps = authentic energy

CHAPTER 6

Conscious breathing

Every physical and emotional state and thought pattern has a corresponding breathing pattern.

> **FELIX'S STORY: BREATHING EASY**
> **Name:** Felix Henderson
> **Age:** 57
> **Condition:** Coronary artery disease, post-traumatic stress
> **Character traits:** Integrity, being passive aggressive
> **Life-changing experiences:** Being in prison; every story that he covered during apartheid
> **Stress catalysts in the last two years:** First myocardial infarction
> **Stress indicators:** Shortness of breath
> **Presentation on energy zone map:** Danger zone

The sound of gunfire rippled through his body, locking his breath in his throat. Blood splattered across the camera lens. It was as if it were raining from hell. 17 June 1992. Boipatong, South Africa. Felix Henderson reporting for the BBC. He didn't need to be there in the midst of anarchy. He had chosen to be. The world needed to hear and see the truth. He remembers the day that he made that commitment. It was 16 June 1976. He was just 19 years old. His cousin had just been shot in Sharpeville. If it wasn't for the brave journalist who captured that heart-wrenching scene, the world would not have known, would not have seen, and Felix may not have been inspired to choose journalism as his vocation.

In those years, the darkest days of apartheid, Felix bore witness to the most harrowing and shocking aspects of humanity. It was only his deep sense of purpose and commitment to the cause that fuelled the courage to continue. In those years, nothing felt safe. No one could be trusted and no one felt safe for him. Whether he was at the scene or smuggling out film reels, Felix was always on high alert. His inner radar system was state of the art. He had developed the ability to sense danger even before the situation became obviously dangerous. For years he had slept with one eye was open and moved like a silent shadow through the stories.

In 1994, when it was all over, Felix felt like he had to leave South Africa. Even though this was an exhilarating time, he was suffocated by the memories. The BBC transferred him to the UK and provided him with a sedate job and a cozy country home just outside central London. Within a year, he booked his flight back home to South Africa, wife and young family in tow. He craved the sunshine, the open skies and the people whose hearts had been stretched open by pain.

Life back home was comfortable. He freelanced for a few publications, and chose to focus on quality time with his family. Weekends were spent in the company of friends and attending his children's school functions. But he carried himself heavily through life, both physically and emotionally. The heart attack, when it came, felt like a jolt back to life for him.

One day Felix caught a glimpse of himself as he passed the mirror in his hallway and saw that he was smiling from the inside. It was as if someone had turned the lights back on somewhere at the back of his hazel eyes, the eyes that have seen more than most.

His mind carried him back to the preceding months and to the day that the pain rippled across his chest and crushed his breath. For a while prior to the 'event', his life had felt as grey as the rebellious strands of hair that stood out like antennae from his head of tight black curls. He got off lightly, with a stent that was inserted into one of his coronary arteries at the time of the angiogram. Somehow, he felt the build up to that moment, when his heart shut down and burst open at the same time. It was not an obvious feeling but rather that his battery was running low. He was finding it difficult to wake up in the morning and his feet felt like heavy weights. He wrote for a few publications but no longer felt engaged with his stories. He was no longer seeing life in full colour.

The myocardial infarction was a call back to life, to passion and meaning. He decided to take action. Felix joined a running club and consulted a dietician. He even considered learning how to meditate. One of his friends had been meditating for years. He had always been skeptical but flirted with the idea of trying it out. That's how he ended up in my consulting room, curious and cautious. He was hoping that I could help guide him in the right direction. As part of Felix's physical examination, we did an assessment of his breathing pattern.

At rest, Felix had a resting respiratory rate of 22 breaths a minute. There was little or no movement of his belly as he breathed. When I asked him to inhale deeply, he did so with great effort as his shoulders shrugged up towards his ears with the muscles in his neck protruding like thick ropes. Felix's breathing pattern revealed his state of health. Years of being in a constant state of hypervigilance had locked his body and breath into an adrenalised mode. His resting breathing rate was higher than was appropriate or healthy.

Every physical and emotional state and thought pattern has a corresponding breathing pattern, which, in turn, has an effect on our physiological state. The breath is the bridge between the mind and body. Felix's breathing was stuck in a pattern reflective of anxiety and fear, his body constantly receiving feedback that he was in danger or in a high-demand situation, even if this was not really the case. Felix was actually 'over breathing' and as a result had been suffering the effects of chronic hyperventilation. Years of being in this adrenalised state was eroding his energy on so many levels and in the process was driving dysfunction even deeper into his cells. His cells were not receiving adequate oxygen as excessive amounts of carbon dioxide was been blown off. We need a certain amount of carbon dioxide in the blood in order to optimise cellular respiration. Carbon dioxide acts as a vasodilator, keeping blood vessels right down the arterial tree open and facilitating the adequate exchange of oxygen at a cellular level. It is also a bronchodilator, helping to keep our airways open too. When we force the exhalations out quickly, we 'blow out' excessive carbon dioxide, and so the carbon dioxide levels in the blood drop and our blood vessels and airways clamp up. This is the reason that we ask people to breathe into a paper bag when they have a panic attack. We are, in fact, asking them to re-breathe carbon dioxide to open up their airways.

Felix was living his life as if it were a long drawn-out panic attack. Even though he had not consciously felt stressed for a long time, his breathing told a different story. And his body believed his breath. His blood vessels had become narrow and tight. Shallow breathing meant that he was not optimising his oxygen intake either. The combination of these factors caused his cells to be chronically starved of oxygen. This in turn set up an inflammatory state in his system. For a long time, Felix had been setting up a perfect breeding ground for chronic illness. His breathing had a lot to do with it. In observing Felix breathe, I noticed that his belly hardly moved, indicating that his diaphragm had become weak from years of disuse. The diaphragm is an amazing parachute-shaped muscle that rests underneath the ribcage, forming the floor of the chest and the roof of the abdomen. As we inhale and the lungs inflate, the diaphragm flattens, pushing the belly out, and as we exhale, the lungs deflate and the diaphragm moves back up into its dome shape. This sheet of muscle is also attached to the lining of the heart (the pericardium), the lining of the lungs (pleura), the spine and even to the large psoas muscle. With every single deep open breath, it's not just the lungs that breathe, the whole body breathes. The body dances to the music of the breath. The bellowing diaphragm massages the liver, spleen, stomach and intestines. Even the heart receives a nourishing massage with each wave of the diaphragm. And Felix with his shallow breathing had been depriving his organs of the opportunity to be massaged and nourished.

All this time, Felix had taken his breath for granted and never considered the impact that his breathing pattern was having on his physical and emotional state. It was only when he joined the running club and required more from his breath that he became aware of how he was breathing. He caught himself in moments, like when he was concentrating on a piece of writing or in a tense moment in a movie, when he unconsciously held his breath. I suggested that we work on some breathing techniques as part of an integrative programme to pave his way to health and to support his authentic energy.

We began with some very simple breath awareness exercises. All he had to do was spend five minutes each morning being a passive observer of his breath, tracking all its details; the temperature of the air as it entered his nostrils, the feeling of his chest expanding and belly rising. By simply turning his attention to his breath at random moments throughout the day, he became more aware of everything else he was experiencing in that moment, including his thought patterns and the habitual patterns of tension in his body.

The next part of the exercise was to hone his focus on the movement of the breath in his belly, a mindfulness technique, which helps to calm a stormy, agitated mind. In his book, *Full Catastrophe Living*, Jon Kabat-Zinn, a well-known mindfulness teacher, speaks about this technique in terms of diving into the stillness of the deep ocean in order to access the peace that resides there. His body drank up the relaxation and energy began to flow through his body again. He became aware of how he was creating unnecessary tension in his system and wasting energy by using the accessory breathing muscles in his neck. After practising this technique for just ten minutes a day for a week, Felix began to notice that he was sleeping better and seemed less irritable and agitated.

The next step was to introduce Felix to simple breathing techniques that he could apply in everyday life situations to manage his energy more effectively. We began with reintroducing him to some simple reflexes that were part of the IPOL's natural energy management system. Sighing is a reflex that happens unconsciously but that we often suppress as it is perceived negatively as a sign of exasperation or irritation. However, it's the body's natural way of releasing tension, slowing down and letting go. This simple sigh of relief is an effective quick recovery loop and a way to take a step back and reboot when life feels overwhelming. Breathing expert Dan Brulé calls this the 'coming home breath', each conscious sigh being an opportunity to tune into ourselves and create a Stillpoint. Next on the menu was the yawn, not a yawn that is swallowed and forced back down by the palm of the hand, but a delicious indulgent yawn that gets the whole body involved. The kind of yawn that invites copious amounts of oxygen into lazy parts of the lungs, that arches the back, gets tears tolling down the cheeks and stretches the arms up to reach for the stars. That kind of yawn instantly refreshes and scoops up energy from the internal natural energy well. Yawning has been widely researched in the scientific community. The effects of yawning are astounding according to recent studies. Yawning cools the brain, stimulates the immune system and triggers the release of endorphins. Felix really struggled with the idea of yawning unashamedly. He noticed how his hand would automatically cover his mouth every time he felt a yawn coming on, even when he was alone; but soon he began to cooperate with his body and enjoy the benefits of a full body yawn every time it was triggered. Just by simply observing his breathing and reconditioning his natural breathing reflexes, Felix began to wake up to the power and potential that resided right under his nose. He wanted to know more.

In order for Felix to re-pattern his breathing, he needed to create a daily breathing practice as if he were learning a new skill. In his case, it was important that we retrain his diaphragm. We did this by getting him to lie on his back with a heavy book on his belly. All he had to do was move the book up and down with his breath, and slow his breathing down as he inhaled for a count of five and exhaled for a count of five. He began and ended every day with this ten-minute breathing practice. Within a couple of weeks, Felix was already feeling the positive effects of conscious breathing. As the diaphragm became stronger with these belly breathing exercises, his lung capacity improved and his blood pressure reduced significantly. He was sleeping better than he ever had and woke up without the alarm jolting him awake as it had for years. He found himself being more present in conversations and more engaged in life.

We also worked with a specific technique of conscious, connected breathing and this became a powerful tool that assisted Felix to release the years of trauma that were locked in his cellular memory. Before long, Felix was experimenting with many breathing techniques and was even getting creative with inventing his own.

When we first started working with the breath, Felix was excited and nervous at the same time. It was almost as if his mind was afraid of what the breath would unleash. And his body was playing along, it being the vault that kept the memories safe and the trauma trapped. He approached the breath slowly and cautiously, first observing it from across the room. They made eye contact and then at last the dance began. Before long, Felix and his breath became best friends. Felix knew that his breath was always there but called on it every time he needed extra support, when he was feeling low, tired, de-energised or when he was in pain. It was even a surprising weight management tool. Breath uncoiled tension from his muscles so that at night he slipped into a deep sleep and it gave him a kick start in the morning. It allowed him to stay focused and soothe away irritability. Breath seemed to freshen up his life and brought colour back into it.

He was amazed at what he was able to achieve just by using the breath. Now, Felix uses his breath in every situation in his life, from dealing with standing in a queue, coming up with creative ideas for a story, winding down before bed, powering up his workout or just simply if he wants to enhance his enjoyment of an experience. Even his libido was back in full force. His wife thought this miraculous. His cardiologist told him to continue whatever he was doing because it was working.

The human system has been exquisitely and precisely designed to maintain a state of equilibrium, despite our ever-changing physiology, emotional state and external environment. The autonomic nervous system has a sophisticated surveillance system that immediately picks up and responds to changes in body temperature, oxygen saturation or life-threatening situations. Signals fire up along the neurological pathways within milliseconds to the appropriate organs and cells, which are called to action to maintain homeostasis. Our breathing is coordinated and directed by the breathing centre in the brain, which is part of our autonomic nervous system. Like our heartbeat, digestion and temperature regulation system, IPOL takes over to manage our breathing.

Our breath is the most exquisite example of innate wisdom in action. It quietly sustains our life force while we get on with the business of our lives. Most of us have never even considered the gift and value of the breath until something comes in the way of its flow.

The effects of conscious breathing

The breathing cycle, the inhale and the exhale, is also the perfect expression of the law of rhythms. With every inhalation, high energy stress response is balanced by the exhalation and recovery state. This can even be measured in our heart rate. When we inhale the heart rate increases slightly, and as we exhale it decreases slightly.

The question you might have is how it is that our breathing becomes so dysfunctional that we have to learn how to breathe again. And what does breathing 'properly' actually mean? As children, our breathing is closest to its natural state, but as we become conditioned and socialised, natural urges and reflexes become suffocated and trapped. Like Felix did, we suffocate our yawns and avoid sighing because of the message it sends to people around us. As our beliefs and perceptions get molded, the more our breath gets jagged and restricted. Being desk bound shuts down our breathing even further. Tension and misalignment in the thoracic spine has a direct impact on the breath too as this is where the back of the diaphragm is attached. Tight clothing is another culprit. Women are often amazed at how much more easily they are able to breathe when they unclip their bras and belts. Even our diet has an impact on the way we breathe. From a mechanical perspective, an over distended stomach pushes up against the diaphragm impeding its movement, but even the kind of food we eat affects our breathing on a biochemical level. Refined carbohydrates, sugars and processed food create an acidic environment in the body. The body's compensatory mechanism to maintain the pH balance is to trigger an increased breathing rate. As in Felix's case, breathing patterns can be yanked out of natural balance by a severe traumatic event or by long-term states of hyperarousal where there's no outlet for the adrenalised energy that builds up over time.

If we are stuck in the danger zone or burnout zone, the breath will reflect that with a habitual pattern of breathing that is shallow, fast and restricted. In addition, our breathing pattern, posture and tone of voice is constantly sending feedback signals to the brain. If the body is sending stress signals to the brain through shallow breath and tight muscles, the brain will react accordingly by feeding adrenalised energy. Eventually, over time, adrenalised energy becomes a habit. However, in just one breath, we can break the cycle of toxic adrenalised energy and shift our energy state.

If that can happen with just one breath, imagine what we are able to achieve if we bring conscious breathing into our daily awareness and integrate it into our lifestyle. But how does this happen? Before I share the techniques with you, it is important to understand the inner workings of the recovery loop. The answer resides in a long and winding nerve called the vagus nerve, the major nerve highway that connects the brain to the body. This interesting nerve unlocks the mystery to the mind-body-and-breath connection. The vagus nerve is part of the parasympathetic rest and digest mode, so when it is activated, the heart rate slows down, our digestive system is stimulated and we feel relaxed and calm. We go into recovery and healing mode. You might have noticed that when you start to relax your tummy will rumble. Most of the fibres of the vagus are responsible for sending signals from the vocal cords, lungs, heart and digestive system back to the brain. Fibres from the vagus nerve wrap around the back of the throat and vocal cords, travel down to circle around the heart and deep into the little air sacs or alveoli in the lungs where they receive signals from the stretch receptors. So each time we take a deep breath, fill our air sacs and release the breath slowly, the vagus nerve is being powerfully stimulated to activate a healing recovery loop.

The long-term aim is to use the breath to strengthen our 'vagal tone', so that instead of the breath being reflective of a stuck adrenalised state, the breath is fluid and adaptive and working with the law of rhythms with every inhale and exhale. The aim is also to develop a deeper awareness of our energy state and to consciously use it to change our state so that it is appropriate and responsive to each situation in which we find ourselves. This is true energy mastery.

What are the qualities of optimum breathing?

- *Open and flowing:* The breathing of a sleeping baby gives us a clue. You might notice how their belly moves and how the breaths occur in a smooth and gentle rhythm. If we stayed connected to this natural way of breathing, our breathing patterns would be unrestricted, open and flowing at rest.
- *Adaptable:* Ideally, the breath adapts to our emotional state and environment in a way that supports our energy instead of depleting it. In times of high demand, such as exercise, the breath deepens and the rate intensifies to meet the metabolic demands of the experience. Once the situation has been dealt with, the body should return to its resting state and the breathing should respond by softening and opening up to a natural gentle flow, supporting our authentic energy. Then the body's self-

- *Right under the nose:* The nose has the perfect architecture to facilitate the delivery of prepared air to the delicate tissues of the lungs. Its aerodynamic design spirals and slows down the inhaled air so that it has enough time to be filtered, warmed and humidified by the mucous membranes in the respiratory tract. Habitual and unconscious mouth breathing at rest is a dysfunctional pattern as this whole mechanism of nasal breathing is bypassed and one becomes susceptible to respiratory infections. However, there are times when using mouth breathing is necessary. These include natural reflexes like yawning, sighing, and when a large amount of air is needed quickly (after being under water for a long time, for example). Notice also that powerful emotions, like laughing, crying, etc., naturally demand mouth breathing.
- *Low and slow:* A maximum healthy respiratory rate is between 10 and 14 breaths per minute at rest. If breathing is faster, as in Felix's case, it could mean that you are chronically hyperventilating. In that case, too much carbon dioxide gets blown off, creating a state of acidity, a breeding ground for chronic illness. Work on breathing techniques where you are consciously slowing the breaths down, imagining that you are breathing from and sending the breaths deep into the pelvis. Consciously training low and slow breathing will reset your breathing to a naturally more slow rhythm.

regulating mechanisms remain intact and untainted by poor posture, stress, emotional baggage and negative thinking.

By now, you may also have the sense that it's not just the lungs that are involved when we breathe. In fact, when breathing optimally, the whole body is involved. With every breath, there is a subtle rocking of the pelvis and movement of the spine that pumps cerebrospinal fluid through it and around the brain. In order for this to happen, it is vital to get the breath moving through the three breathing spaces in your body: the lower breathing space is located between the tip of the tailbone to the navel; the middle breathing space rests between the navel and the nipple line; and the upper breathing space lies between the nipple line and collarbones.

From Felix's story we can see that breathing is far more than breathing in oxygen and breathing out carbon dioxide. In fact, breathing is the most powerful, simple and underrated energy management tool that exists. Breath and energy go hand in hand. The ability to master the breath offers the mastery of energy and of life itself. The breath ignites IPOL into a vital and blazing source of energy that flows through every organ, muscle and cell. More than simply delivering oxygen to the cells, life force rides on the back of the breath waking up the mind and body to its full potential.

Some benefits of optimum breathing:
- Supports detoxification on a cellular level
- Improves focus and concentration
- Breaks cycle of adrenalised energy
- Improves sleep
- Tool for anti-ageing
- Enhances sports performance
- Supports emotional intelligence
- Assists in managing pain
- Helps to break down negative habits and patterns
- Strengthens the immune system
- Reduces blood pressure

Before we can start using specific breathing techniques, we first have to learn to connect with our natural breathing and establish a relationship with it. Get into a habit of turning your awareness to your breath throughout the day. Notice how you are breathing when you are typing an email, engaging in conversation, sitting in traffic, feeling overwhelmed or feeling calm and happy. As soon as you become aware of how you are breathing, you will automatically become aware of your posture, thoughts, reactions, habits and patterns. Breath awareness is also the foundation of mindfulness meditation practice, which you can use as a recovery loop at the beginning and end of your day. Sit in a comfortable position feeling your feet on the floor. Simply notice that you are breathing. Feel the air in your nostril and the feeling of the breath rising and falling as you inhale and exhale. Let this be the anchor of your awareness. As soon as you notice your mind wandering, don't get frustrated or judge your thoughts, simply bring your attention back to the breath, its character and how it's feeling and moving in your body. You can begin by doing this for five minutes at a time and build up to 15 or 20 minutes.

Balancing breath or coherent breathing

This is a great technique to balance your energy by equalising the energy and relaxation response with the inhale and exhale. It effectively brings down cortisol levels, stimulates the immune system and balances homeostasis. Use it at the beginning of the day as part of your morning ritual after your breath awareness practice or as a stand-alone technique. It is also helpful to use when you are feeling overwhelmed, stressed and anxious. Lie down or sit in a comfortable position. Keeping your shoulders relaxed, deepen and slow down the inhalation, breathing slowly from low down in your belly all the way to the top of your lungs for a count of five seconds. Exhale very slowly and completely for a count of five seconds. Breathe continuously without gaps or pauses between the inhale and exhale. David O'Hare, in his book *365, Heart Coherence* suggests doing this technique three times a day for five minutes at a time.

Breathing for relaxation

Throughout this book, we have been exploring the idea of mastering energy through the skill of relaxation, recovery and renewal. We also now understand the science behind how it can be used to achieve this. The key lies in the exhale, the 'action' of letting go. Yawning and sighing are quick, effective ways to activate 'micro' recovery loops throughout the day between meetings, phone calls and other tasks. If you are feeling particularly wound up or anxious, deepen the relaxation response by spending more time on the exhalation. For example, inhale for a count of five and exhale slowly for a count of ten. Find a ratio that works for you. The idea is to double the time of the exhalation. If you would like to deepen your relaxation even further, you can hold the breath for a few seconds before you exhale. For example, inhale for a count of five. Hold the breath for a count of five, exhale slowly and completely for a count of eight. Continue for five to ten minutes.

Breathing for energy

Whenever we need an energy boost, we can harness the energy response and use it in a focused and conscious way. For example, while exercising, or when we need confidence before a presentation or interview, focus on the inhalation.

Lengthen the inhalation by 'doubling' the inhalation, drawing the breath into your belly and chest, feeling the expansion in three dimensions. Breath expert Dan Brulé describes this as 'charging up the heart'. Practise how to power breathe, which is a slightly more advanced and very powerful technique that is very energising and relaxing at the same time. It is also known as '20 connected breaths'. This one involves using your mouth to breathe. Take a long deep slow inhalation, filling your lungs right to the top. Imagine that you are sucking the breath through a thick straw. Let the exhale drop out like a sigh of relief. Keep breathing in this way with no gaps or pauses between the breaths 20 times. Let every fifth breath be a longer one. Begin each morning with this technique and practise this at least three times during the day for a power boost.

Get playful with your breath and use it in a way that supports your energy in every aspect of your life. Visit www.breathtechapp.com to download a free app created by Dan Brulé and myself for some great guided practices through eight different paths from health to sports and business performance. Our breath moves, flows and adapts itself under the radar of our conscious awareness and yet, when we come alive to it, notice it and harness it, it becomes the very force that shifts us from operating at baseline level to expanding and growing in ways we never imagined possible.

> Energy Formula
> *Breath awareness + conscious breathing (relaxation and energy)*
> *= authentic energy*

CHAPTER 7

Exercise

Like everything else, creating the changes in the way that we work with our bodies requires a multidimensional approach.

> **NIDARA'S STORY: FLOW WITHIN FORM**
> **Name:** Nidara Mia
> **Age:** 47
> **Character traits:** Fearlessness, sacrificing for others at her own expense
> **Life-changing experiences:** Being part of the anti-apartheid struggle
> **Stress catalysts in last two years:** Extensive travel for her UN job
> **Stress indicators:** Fatigue, inability to 'switch off the mind'
> **Presentation on energy zone map:** Burnout zone

The American Airlines jet lifted off the runway and made a tangent towards the sun. The rain drops on the pigeonhole window blurred the Manhattan skyline before it faded and vanished. Nidara rummaged through her handbag, extracted an eye mask and shut out the world. She had just closed a chapter of her life and had no energy to feel the loss.

The last three years working as a policy maker at the UN office in

New York had been exhilarating and impactful. On a professional level it was a period of growth and expansion. She lifted the ceiling of what she thought she was capable of. Her work on gender equality had taken her from Accra to Addis Ababa, from Beirut to Berlin. She had advised policy makers, inspired fresh ideas and supported governments despite opposition, defiance and calcified thinking. She had always thrived on taking herself to the edge and showing her metal. It was how she was wired. Defiance was in her blood. She had fought against apartheid in South Africa. She had married a black man despite the wishes of her conservative Muslim family. Having risen to the rank of advocate, she had worked in a fractured South African government justice system. She was hoping to find more fulfilment at the UN. After three intense years, she knew that her time in New York had come to an end. It was time to come home, back to South Africa. Back to herself.

Nidara had been experiencing incapacitating fatigue for a long time. She could almost predict the pattern of her energy dips. Interspersed with the long periods of fatigue, she would feel an occasional surge of energy in response to an idea, inspiration or achieved goal, but mostly she had to muster it up. She was familiar with the daily battle between her mind and duvet in the morning; the relative rise of energy between midmorning and 3pm and the deep dip in the afternoons. She knew that she would take a few days to find balance after travelling and that that time was becoming progressively longer. She was acutely aware of her body's signals. She had created her own strategy to cope. She knew what to do to keep going. She knew what supplements to take and the right doctor to see who sold liquid energy through vitamin drips. She squeezed in the odd yoga class between meetings and travel, and felt consoled that she did so much walking. Life in New York demanded it.

Nidara's health strategies kept her functioning at baseline. She dealt with her symptoms as they rose with deft practicality. She knew it wasn't good enough. Her family knew too. They were able to read her signals and found a way to adapt to her erratic patterns. Her son, a wise and intuitive nine-year-old, was quick to point out when she needed a 'time out'. This is how Nidara navigated her life and career. It was an energy roller coaster. Her lifestyle was in stark contrast to that of her husband's, with whom she had once shared a racy lifestyle, but he was taking advantage of taking space and time out for himself in New York. A respected human rights lawyer in his own right, Nidara's husband Mpho enjoyed New York's cultural life, spending time with their son and lecturing occasionally at the University of New York.

When Mpho was offered a position to head up an exciting project back home in Johannesburg, Nidara encouraged it. The thought of returning home was comforting. On the long flight back from New York, through the shadows of her mind, Nidara began to craft a vision for her new life. A life coloured with space and soul. Right there, among the clouds and the stars, she decided that her life and her health would be her next project until she felt ready to decide on her next career move. The butterflies in her belly had the shades of both excitement and anxiety.

For the first time since finishing school, Nidara finally would have the space and will to rest, recover and envision the next part of her life and career. She had it all mapped out. She knew exactly how she was going to implement her plan.

Nidara practically leapt from the tarmac to the treadmill. A few days after arriving back in Johannesburg she had signed up at the local gym and found a personal trainer. Project 'Perfect Health' was underway. With the same fiery determination with which she approached everything in her life, Nidara was at the gym religiously at 6am every morning. She trained six days a week, determined to drop 15 kilograms quickly. The excitement of starting her new personal project ignited a newfound energy in her. Funky gym gear found a space in her wardrobe among her business suits. Nidara had been surviving on adrenalised energy for a very long time. It had impacted the functioning of her thyroid gland which slowed down her metabolism. Subcutaneous fat deposits around her waist were linked to insulin resistance, which in turn caused havoc with her glucose levels. Her high cholesterol levels were linked to low thyroid hormones.

As part of Nidara's perfect health plan, she scheduled a session with a dietician, who designed a strict protein-based eating plan to support the weight loss in combination with her training. Portions had to be weighed and measured for every meal with precisely the right proportion of fat, protein and minimal carbohydrate. It felt good to be control.

A month into her training programme, Nidara scheduled her routine weigh in; her body fat percentage had increased. So had her weight. She was more tired than ever and felt burdened by her health restoration programme. She felt that she could no longer trust her body; that it was working against her. She had reached the tipping point, on the brink of falling into the burnout zone. With fierce retaliation, Nidara made a bee line back to the gym, cranked up the speed on the treadmill and sprinted furiously through her pounding heart, burning chest and trembling thighs.

One afternoon, Nidara collapsed on her bed, dehydrated and limp. The room spun around her, nausea seeped into every cell. Emotion came like a tsunami. She cried a lifetime of tears. Tears of grief for the loss of a newly found life and a circle of friends, tears of sadness for all the suffering to which she bore witness. Tears of uncertainty, not knowing where her life path was leading, tears of anger that she had failed herself and tears of gratitude as her son walked into the room and put his head in her lap without saying a word.

The next day, Nidara paid me a visit. It was wonderful to see her after her return from New York. Nidara was one of the first patients that I had treated for burnout in my early years as an integrated practitioner. Working with her helped shape my understanding of burnout, the psychobiological factors involved and the principles that govern energy. It was disconcerting to see her fragility and disillusionment. Her almond-shaped eyes lacked their usual sparkle, her mocha skin missed its rosy kiss. The dam of feelings that were unleashed in her tears the day before were still evident under her unconvincing smile. Nidara expressed her frustration with measured eloquence. Why had her body fat percentage shot up despite all the effort she was putting into the training? Why had her energy levels dropped so dramatically after her workouts to the point of an emotional breakdown? She shared that she had lost all enjoyment from eating. She was just going through the motions, and followed all the rules of eating the 'right way'. There was a momentary glint in her eyes as her rebellious nature broke through. Her connection with her body and desire to do things differently was beginning to emerge.

What stood out most starkly in my conversation with Nidara was that her exercise regime was working against her rather than for her. She approached her suggested workouts with the same zeal that she dealt with everything else in her life. It had to be done right, perfectly, by the book. In the process, she became her own greatest enemy. Nidara had been experiencing challenges with managing her energy for a long time. Through our work together over the years, she had developed a solid foundation of understanding of her body and her warning signs for burnout. Despite this, her old patterns of striving, pushing and achieving had shown up in her health restoration plan to her own detriment.

Before we took any further steps to design Nidara's energy recovery plan, it was imperative that she recognised and owned her 'old pattern' and that in order for her to achieve sustainable health and energy, her perception of a 'healthy lifestyle' and exercise would have to be re-evaluated. We spent some time chatting about cortisol, the stress hormone that often gets such a bad rap. I reminded her that cortisol is not all bad. In fact, if the body didn't produce cortisol, we would find it impossible to get out of bed in the morning. Cortisol is naturally released in the blood stream in a particular pattern throughout the day, giving us energy when we need it most, and helping us to wind down as we prepare to rest and recover. It spikes when we have a need for energy in a high-demand situation and falls again when we have used up the energy it has provided through the chain of chemical reactions.

It was also clear that Nidara had a typical 'fire personality' – sharp-witted, fierce and dynamic. In her early life, her physique reflected that too. Her body burned everything she consumed quickly. Her metabolism was a furnace. While she had a natural

Pitta (Fire) personality, her body had become more sluggish as her prolonged high levels of cortisol took its toll on her physiology and energy.

The way that she had been exercising since her return was, in fact, causing havoc with her already compromised adrenal system. Nidara had been in the danger zone for a long time and was beginning to dip into the burnout zone, and on further investigation it became evident why her body had responded to the extreme exercise the way it had. Nidara would arrive at the gym either at the crack of dawn, so that she would make it back home in time to take her son to school, or at the end of the day when she had worked through her 'to do' list of setting up their new home. She would hop onto the treadmill and begin at the highest speed she could manage to warm up and save time. In her workouts, Nidara pushed herself beyond the pain of over-exertion and injury. Like everything else, she relied on her strong mind to get her through her routine. Often this was beyond what her body could deal with. She was working out almost every day with no recovery time.

By the time she arrived at the gym, her cortisol levels were already peaked from planning the activities of the day. The level that she began working out with spiked her cortisol even further, chipping away at her already compromised adrenal system. This, of course, had a ripple effect on the rest of her endocrine system. The cells in her body were becoming less and less sensitive to her insulin and thyroid hormones and thus less efficient. The demands of cortisol were causing her progesterone levels to plummet, driving her towards premature menopause. Exercising in this way was also impacting her immune system, which was struggling to produce the antibodies and immunoglobulins needed to keep infections at bay, and thus she found that she was catching every virus that did its rounds. Although she always felt her pulse racing, she was unaware of what her actual heart rate was during her workouts and instead of progressively building up her heart rate, she waited for the burn in her chest as the signal to stop. Even though she was not formally working since returning to South Africa, rushing was still her modus operadi, so she usually gave the post workout stretch a skip. It seemed like such a waste of time.

Nidara was able to smile at herself as she recognised her 'all or nothing' behaviour playing out with her exercise too. Just a few months ago, she was barely exercising at all, and hadn't even given herself the opportunity to build up an awareness of how her body was responding to the workouts. It didn't occur to her that her fitness level and strength needed to be built up. She hadn't even considered the possibility that she was, in fact, driving the burnout even deeper through the way she was training.

Before we embarked on the process of crafting a more sustainable and realistic exercise regime, Nidara and I reflected on her relationship with exercise in her life.

'I was never the champion athlete at school. Just mediocre, never quite making the bar in high jump or hitting the mark in the long jump. Always almost. My relationship with my body came through yoga and some dance. Non-competitive, flowing and feminine. Swimming fitted into that category. That came more naturally. I guess this was a combination of nature and nurture. I grew up in a family that was more academic than sporty, and sport wasn't something that was encouraged or valued as it was in other families. When sports no longer become compulsory, I gravitated towards my comfort zone of yoga, a place where I could explore my physicality in a non-threatening way.

'However, through my experience of various yoga practices, styles and teachers I became starkly aware of how easy it is to bring the element of ego and competitiveness into the realm of yoga. And that it is possible to cause harm, be aggressive in yoga too. However, it always niggled at me that my cardiovascular fitness was something that was important to work on, because of my family history of cardiovascular disease and the fact that I was getting older. And, of course, vanity is always a great motivator for change, but even that wasn't impetus enough. That day on the flight back home I knew it was time to get my butt on that bicycle and bulk up the biceps.'

I referred Nidara to Dorian Cabral and his wife Leigh, two highly experienced trainers who work with many burnt out executives. They knew this pattern of exercise well. In fact, they had seen many examples of people who had caused more harm than good through their exercise programmes. The first thing that Dorian suggested was that Nidara purchase a heart rate monitor so that she was able to carefully monitor her heart rate as she was training and, more importantly, this was a way for Nidara to monitor herself and keep her awareness and focus on what the body was experiencing as she was exercising. Nidara spent most of the first training session lying on a mat on her back as Leigh guided her into a body- and breath-awareness exercise. She was made to become more aware of how her body was orientated, where she was feeling tension and how she was breathing. Initially her mind fought against this seemingly pointless exercise. How was lying on a mat going to get her to lose 15 kg?

The point was that Nidara could only move forward after she had established a deeper awareness of her body, her breath and sense of proprioception. Once this was in place, she could then use the breath to power her energy more efficiently in the workouts. Leigh helped her to develop the awareness of when she was habitually overusing her upper trapezius and upper body (primary and secondary muscles) in order to compensate for weak core muscles. She began to see how areas of weakness in her body were being compensated for by other parts. She realised how all the years of sitting at a desk hunched over a computer caused her body to contract into a stooped posture that was impacting on her breathing and the way she moved. Her chronically tight jaw was directly connected to the tightness in her lower back through the big psoas muscle that connects the hip to the lower back. Nidara had developed the typical round-shouldered posture often seen in people who spend hours stooped over desks. This in turn fed the cycle of adrenalised energy even more furiously.

Next she hopped on the bicycle and, again, Nidara had to begin at a very low intensity and speed, at the same time carefully watching what was happening to her heart rate and internal state. This was how she had to start every training session, with warming up for 15 to 20 minutes, increasing the speed every two minutes to maintain homeostasis (state of internal balance) and ensuring that her heart rate remained at 60% of her maximum heart rate. In this way, she would avoid the cortisol spike and her body would be given time to adjust to the increasing intensity of the workouts. 'The workout is in the warm up' was her trainer's mantra.

In the first few months of her 'new training regime', the focus for Nidara was to stabilise, neutralise and mobilise the smaller muscle groups through functional training. In this way, she strengthened her core, working with specific muscle groups and building her sense of balance and proprioception. Every workout session ended with 10 minutes of breathing and deep stretching, to activate the parasympathetic nervous system (rest and recover mode) and reestablish homeostasis before heading back into the world.

She watched as her body slowly became sculpted into a new curvaceous shape, but more than that, she began sleeping soundly and woke up feeling rested and refreshed after a night's sleep. The alarm on her smartphone became a redundant app. Her relationship with food also shifted dramatically. Her body began to crave more fresh vegetables and protein from fish and chicken. Nuts felt like a far more appealing snack than a chocolate bar. She was amazed at how IPOL had woken up and that she was able to listen and act on what she was becoming aware of. It was as if her cells celebrated every time she ate something fresh and wholesome. She had finally raised the white flag on herself and succumbed to the wisdom of her body.

Over a few months, Nidara established a manageable routine of functional training, light weight training, cardiovascular exercise and yoga. Between her training sessions, which were focused and structured, she allowed her cardiovascular exercises to become fun, spontaneous and creative. This took the form of Sunday hikes with the family, riding bikes or going to a dance class. Yoga was still something she enjoyed, and more so now that her core strength had improved so dramatically.

For Nidara, exercise moved from being something she feared and dreaded to becoming a great adventure. She became fascinated with the inner mechanics of the body, particularly with the idea that every joint and muscle from the sole of the foot to the back of the head is connected by an 'inner skin', called the fascia. The skeleton would be nothing but a loose bag of bones if it was not connected through this tough and elastic tissue. She noticed that on days when she spent a long time sitting, her hips would feel contracted and her shoulders and jaw would tense up. She could literally feel the ripple of tension through her body. Even the diaphragm which is part of the fascia seized up on these days and tugged at her breathing pattern.

Her awareness of her energy became so finely tuned that she would feel the difference in the quality of her energy after a gym training session and a yoga session, which was fascinating since we now know that different kinds of exercise promote the release of different kinds of chemicals. Running felt like she was freeing locked up stress from her body, while resistance training connected her to her inner warrior, making her feel strong and confident. And after a yoga class she felt a heightened state of natural energy, centred and aware.

A year down the line, Nidara was feeling stronger, fitter and more energised than she'd ever been. Surprisingly her weight was no longer an obsession. Far more important to her was the way she was feeling. Needless to say, Nidara lost weight. Her eating habits were driven by the feeling of health and energy rather than weight loss. Her belly fat had practically disappeared, she had dropped two dress sizes and she developed the confident stride of a jaguar. When we looked at her blood tests, there was no doubt that Nidara had successfully created a whole new body. She had, in fact, created a whole new body–mind system. This was reflected in her insulin levels that had normalised, as had her thyroid function.

Nidara had sparked up a whole new neural pathway from her conscious mind to every cell in her body. She had upgraded the software in her subconscious mind that was previously driven by striving and disconnection from her body. It was far more than simply just exercising that got her to this point. Exercise had moved from being just another item on her 'to do' list to an experience that required an acknowledgement of old mental programming and fears. It was an experience that supported mindfulness, and honouring of energy cycles, and ultimately long-term sustainable health and energy.

Exercising for authentic energy

Exercise is an absolute fundamental pillar of body intelligence and, more importantly, how we exercise will determine whether it is supporting or surreptitiously depleting our energy. Like our relationship with food, our relationship with exercise and the way we connect with the physical body is layered and complex. It is shaped by early life experiences, as well as self-imposed and societal-based ideas of perfection. Few of us are comfortable and completely at ease within our bodies. We either loathe it and disconnect from it, or place so much emphasis on the perfect external image that we become overly identified with it. In both cases, we become shut off from the experience of 'being in the body' and listening to its subtle cues, messages and guidance. We end up judging, abusing, punishing and getting frustrated with it. Mostly we take it for granted.

When we perceive exercise from the perspective of image or escapism, we are already creating a rocky foundation and losing out on its real benefits. Like everything else, creating the changes in the way that we work with our bodies requires a multidimensional approach. New neural pathways are created when the mind and body are connected. One needs the other.

It is widely accepted that being physically active is the single most important thing that we can do to maintain our health and energy. We see how exercise literally changes the structure and function of our cells. Thousands of studies have been done on the effects and benefits of exercise. Some of them are:

- Boosts mental performance and cognitive function.
- Reduces the symptoms of depression and anxiety by having an effect on the neurotransmitters like dopamine and serotonin.
- Strengthens the immune system and its ability to fight off certain cancers.

- Reduces inflammation in the system.
- Improves cells' sensitivity to insulin and thyroid hormones.
- Reduces belly fat, reducing the risk of cardiovascular disease and metabolic syndrome.
- The science of epigenetics is showing that exercise switches off inherited genes that cause illness.
- Weight-bearing or resistance training elicits the testosterone response and increases bone density which is important for both men and women.
- Aerobic exercise and endurance training increases energy levels by increasing muscular efficiency and aerobic fitness. Running or jogging gives us the opportunity to be outdoors in the fresh air and natural light. It also elicits the cortisol response, so be aware of this if you are in danger zone or burnout zone.
- Stretching with modalities like yoga opens the flow of energy through the body. Pilates builds core strength and also tones and balances the intrinsic muscles, setting them up as primary movers. Slow mindful exercise sharpens the awareness of the inside of your body and subtle sensory indicators. This will allow us to be more attuned to the body's status.

We all know the basic pillars of health. What we don't think about is that it's not what we do but how we do it that will determine its effect on our life. Exercise can only support and restore our energy and health if we use it mindfully and not reactively. If we are using exercise as a way to tune out, distract ourselves or focus on the exterior benefits, it has the potential to do more harm than good, as it feeds the monster of adrenalised energy.

Here are some guidelines around how you can make exercise an enjoyable and energising experience. Not everyone needs to or has the resources to have a skilled personal trainer; however, the following may be helpful to keep in mind when creating your exercise programme.

A question of time: Time is often the greatest perceivable obstacle when it comes to exercise. This is the biggest false belief that we have. In fact, exercise gives us time as we become far more efficient and effective with everything else that we do by supporting higher levels of energy, focus and concentration. To reframe the belief of 'there's no time', we have to see the importance of exercising as a primary way to invest in our energy.

Invest in yourself: Don't open yourself up to the debate of whether you should or shouldn't exercise. Break out of the habit of procrastination. Get a partner, trainer, join a class. Find something that works for you, get an accountability partner and keep going until it becomes an entrenched behaviour.

Tired or wired: Often we can't get ourselves into an exercise routine because the fatigue in itself is an obstacle, but in making the time to build on your strength, endurance and flexibility, exercise will give you all the energy you need. If you are already in the burnout zone, start slowly with supervision, progressively building up strength. Slow exercise like Tai Chi, Pilates or yoga is a good way to start. If you are feeling wired, be careful not to over exercise. How do you know if you are over exercising? Be awake to the way exercise is making you feel. You should be left with a feeling of 'calm energy'. Check in to see if you are not exercising to release excessive amounts of euphoria-inducing endorphins or a more subtle feeling of strength, energy and alignment.

Balance vs integration: For the purposes of this chapter I am using the words movement and exercise interchangeably. Movement shouldn't just be another item on the 'to do' list, but rather integrated into your day just as your meals are. Take every opportunity to move and stand, for example, standing and walking to meetings, walking to someone's desk instead of sending an email, take the stairs, etc. Make conscious choices to move. Use exercise as a way to move, breathe, practise mindfulness, connect with your body and be in nature.

Free the fascia: The body is reflective of our lifestyle, beliefs, thought patterns, attitudes and emotions. The fascia, which is our second skeleton, holds habitual patterns of movement and ultimately shows up in our postural pattern. A tight fascia traps the free flow of blood, lymph and subtle energy through the body and can become a massive energy drainer as a result. Stretching mindfully through forms of exercise like yoga is an effective way to free yourself from your fascial trap as it opens up and hydrates the fascial sheath. Other ways to free the fascia is through regular deep tissue massage, physiotherapy and chiropractic treatments. More specialised systems to repattern the posture through fascial release include the Alexander technique, rolfing, Feldenkrais and postural integration.

Tailor it: As mentioned numerous times in this book, there is no 'one size fits all' approach to one's journey to wellbeing. It is helpful to have basic guidelines and to be aware of the benefits of different kinds of movement and exercise. But only you can determine what kind of exercise will be most supportive of your body type, constitution, lifestyle and needs. You can only do this when you start to develop a deeper awareness of your body and cultivate your relationship with it. For example, a much adrenalised person in the danger zone would benefit from more strength and resistance training while limiting cardiovascular exercise to no more than 20 minutes day. They would probably find the slower pace of yoga challenging but would greatly benefit from the restorative and centring effects of it. Cardiovascular exercise combined with strength and conditioning training would be most suitable for someone who is overweight and who feels bloated and sluggish.

Mix it up: Use your body to constantly spark up new neural pathways. When the body experiences a new movement, a new connection sparks up in the brain. The more you repeat the exercise, the more you will develop the part of the brain that regulates that movement. By practising the new movements, you are constantly creating new connections and in the process you are able to shape a whole new brain!

Exercise is a wonderful opportunity to practise being present and mindful. Use the time to tune in rather than zone out. Many of us use exercise as a form of escapism, or to get high from an endorphin rush, which is what leads to injuries and chronic wear and tear. Before starting your session or class, take inventory of your energy reserves. If you are exhausted when you start, and you overexert, you will exhaust yourself further. Rest a bit before starting, take some deep breaths, ground yourself and build up slowly.

Pace yourself. Your personality/energy signature will be reflected in the way you exercise. There is a perfect pace that will energise you. Find your pace that challenges growth at the edge of your comfort zone but at the same time works within your body's energy capacity. To find this edge, observe your rate of exercise, habitual overuse of certain muscles, core strength, alignment, flow of energy, thoughts and images.

Like breathing, the way we exercise is often how we do everything else in our lives. Your exercise mat and treadmill can be a good training ground for life.

Energy Formula
Warm up x (strength + endurance + flexibility) x wind down
= authentic energy

CHAPTER 8

Tapping into nature

We need to create an awareness of the role of nature in our lives.

> **ISABELLA'S STORY: THE ART OF RECOVERY**
> **Name:** Isabella Duarte
> **Age:** 39
> **Character traits:** Sense of humour, ability to engage and connect with people, Chutzpah, impulsivity
> **Life-changing experiences:** Working with the gangs, trip to India, illness of her uncle
> **Stress catalysts in the last two years:** Juggling the work of two businesses, corporate job and motherhood
> **Stress indicators:** Jaded view of life, lack of exercise, fatigue
> **Presentation on energy zone map:** Danger zone

Isabella steps across the reception floor of the consulting company where she is employed. She places one high-heeled foot in front of the other while balancing the weight of her lap top bag and oversized handbag across both shoulders. She has bigger problems, but none as crucial as this one. The left heel of her favourite pair of shoes is wobbling, threatening to fall off and send her flying through reception at any given moment. It's her favourite pair and the only one that matches her dress. The only dress that fits when she's premenstrual and feeling bloated. Somehow she makes it to the lift and to her cubicle in the middle of the open-plan office. A sad-looking, spiky succulent plant on her desk stares at her, looking as dehydrated as she feels. It's a good thing that she doesn't need to do much walking today. She's office bound and in meetings all day. It's been another week of navigating traffic, drafting proposals, meeting deadlines, supporting her mother whose brother is undergoing chemotherapy and spending quality time with her eight-year-old son who is on school holiday. She's running late for a meeting with some of the directors and an important client. She has no choice but to walk deliberately and with full awareness of every step. It's a weirdly refreshing experience to be slowing down, even if it's by default.

Grateful to have arrived safely behind the boardroom table, Isabella tunes into the meeting, and hones in on what is being negotiated. Her attention switches to her client who is sitting across the table with the window creating a frame behind her. Isabella has had many heated meetings with this stoic woman with strong sculpted features. Usually, this tough and astute business woman would never miss a single word or nuance in a meeting. Today, her chair is swivelled away from the table and her neck is tilted. Her shoulder is arched slightly towards the back of the chair. She slides it a few millimetres back until the rays of the sun hit the nape of her neck, where a few strands of hair have fallen from her loose chignon. Her eyes soften and breath deepens. It's as if she's feeling the sun on her skin for the very first time. It's a sacred Stillpoint moment, and within it, Isabella sees herself and remembers.

Isabella grew up on a farm on the banks of the Crocodile River tributary outside Johannesburg near an area known as the Cradle of Humankind. She spent carefree days climbing trees and playing hide and seek behind the rocks and in the cowshed. Her mother was the quintessential matriarch, salt of the earth, open-minded and rebellious. Her dad was a free spirit and courageous entrepreneur. She ate freshly laid eggs for breakfast and once in a while the turkey became a delicious roast. She lived in harmony with nature's rhythms. Living close to nature informed her understanding of life. The sun energised and refreshed her, the moon reminded her of magic and every star was a dream of a future that she couldn't wait to create.

Her flecked green eyes speak of energy, intensity and a deep need for impact. She is driven by her convictions and passion to support people to fulfil their potential. Her job at the consulting firm provides her with the opportunity to do just that. Accepting this position has meant that she had to move off the farm and closer to the office. She was hoping that spending less time in traffic would mean more time for herself and things she loved to do, but it didn't quite turn out like that. Six years into this job and her career has taken off. She is valued by the organisation and her efforts are recognised and rewarded.

If only she felt the same about the rest of her life. Isabella and her husband have been struggling to conceive for the last six years, since Damian, her son, was two years old. It has become a great source of frustration and anxiety. Her menstrual cycle has become erratic and she has noticed her levels of irritability mounting. She's been experiencing headaches, joint pain and a constant low-grade nausea. Emotionally she feels fragile and tearful, which in turn makes her anxious about being perceived as weak and out of control. Her skin is breaking out around her chin and her eyes constantly feel dry and strained. All her energetic resources are channelled into her work where she ensures that she remains sharp, focused and on top of her game, but her body seems to have lost its rhythm in the process. She struggles to fall asleep and wakes up numerous times at night. She's never used an alarm but now she's finding that she's become dependent on it and hits the snooze button more than once before dragging herself out of bed.

Moving into the city required a radical mind shift for Isabella. For most of her life, she thrived off the unpolluted country air and eating fresh vegetables picked from the garden. Her city apartment was slick but synthetic. She felt suffocated in her cubicle in the open-plan office with its recycled air and lights that hurt her eyes.

There were aspects of living in the city that Isabella really enjoyed. She loved the theatre and looked forward to trying out the quirky restaurants and coffee shops with her close friends. City life was exciting but over-stimulating. She found it difficult to switch off from the fast pace even if it was not necessary or appropriate. What she chose as relaxing activities were actually driving the 'adrenalised' state even further. Isabella was emphatic about keeping fit and ensured that she got to the gym at least three times a week. Life was good but often she yearned for the simplicity of just sitting in the garden staring up at a sky full of stars.

From the outset it was clear that even though Isabella was highly efficient at work, her body was functioning in the danger zone. Her physical symptoms began when she moved into the city. It was then that she had become disconnected from nature, a source of energy that had always been fundamental in her life. In the process, Isabella had lost the natural oscillation between high intensity periods of life and work and deep periods of rest, which living in the country and close to nature facilitated. The greatest impact was on her endocrine system. The infertility was just the tip of the iceberg of a story that went far back.

All the information gathered from Isabella's physical examination and blood tests indicated that her endocrine system was taking strain. Communication between her organs and endocrine system had broken down, sending confusing messages to the body, brain and pituitary gland, the master controller of the endocrine system that is situated within the brain. The combination of exposure to artificial lighting, disrupted sleep patterns and prolonged high levels of stress hormones were all contributing factors. Both progesterone and cortisol are made from the same mother hormone, DHEA. Because Isabella's body was producing more cortisol in response to stress, less DHEA was available to make progesterone and this is one of the reasons that her fertility was becoming compromised.

Based on what we established through Isabella's story, examination and investigations, we decided that before embarking on any form of sophisticated treatment, we would begin with the basics and work on reestablishing Isabella's natural rhythms and cycles using nature. We began Isabella's programme with prescribing 20 minutes of natural sun exposure every day. Practically this meant taking a jog or walk around her suburb instead of on the treadmill or simply sitting on her balcony to soak up the morning rays while having breakfast. I encouraged her to plant some flowers and grow some herbs in planters, to remind her of how little is needed to encourage the growth of life. The programme also entailed at least three hours of being in nature every weekend. This could take the form of going on a picnic, going on a hike or going mountain biking with the family. I encouraged her to walk barefoot on grass. The feet contain a rich network of nerves and acupuncture points. Walking barefoot picks up electrons from the earth's surface, which neutralises free radicals and activates the parasympathetic nervous system. I recommended that she get out of the city for a long weekend at least every four months for a deeper nature immersion or nature therapy.

In Isabella's case, it was important that we went back to the root cause of the infertility in order to treat it and thus my reason for prescribing nature therapy was twofold. Firstly, I was using nature as a way to activate deep recovery and replenishment of her energy. We all know the familiar feeling of inner stillness and soothing that nature facilitates. We generally feel calmer, thoughts are clearer and we breathe deeper. When we're in a beautiful natural environment, we feel free to take in more of life and we are simply more present and in the moment. Walking barefoot on the grass, even sitting under a tree, are examples of powerful recovery loops. Secondly, I was prescribing nature therapy to reestablish the balance of her endocrine system specifically through the sun. The sun is a life-giving source of energy and nourishment. When we are exposed to adequate amounts of natural sunlight, our circadian rhythm is regulated through the hormone melatonin, which is released through the pineal gland, and vitamin D, which is vital for so many aspects of health, is converted to its active form. Sunlight travels along the optic nerve to the pineal gland in the brain and is stimulated to release the 'feel good' hormones serotonin and dopamine, and other neurotransmitters that regulate our brain chemistry. This, in turn, activates a chain reaction of communication through the glands of the endocrine system, which all work as a synchronised system. As in Isabella's case, if one aspect of the system is disrupted by something as simple as inadequate light exposure, it has a serious knock-on effect without us even realising it.

Shift work, regular travel across time zones and even working in offices where there is no natural sunlight can cause disruption of the entire neuroendocrine system, which can affect fertility, immune system function and the endocrine system. In fact, prolonged disruption of the circadian rhythm is now thought to be an independent risk factor for cancer.

Isabella was surprised at how quickly her body responded to the simple changes that she was making. It was as if her body was remembering its ancient knowing and rewarded her for the gentle support she was offering it. She was calmer and more focused at work. She felt inspired to have fresh flowers in her home and put plants on her desk at work, and even introduced colour and creativity into her wardrobe of greys and blacks. She realised that her sleep was becoming restorative but, most importantly, Isabella was beginning to realise what a refreshed relaxation felt like and was more conscious when she was feeling 'inappropriate' adrenalised energy. In this way, she was becoming savvier around how to use her energy more efficiently. For Isabella, seeing nature in action was a reminder to honour her own cycles of activity and rest. She began to enjoy this 'new' way of living so much that falling pregnant no longer felt like a priority. Four months later her pregnancy test came back positive.

Nature and IPOL

We began this book talking about IPOL, the intelligent pulse of life; the pulse of energy that is intrinsic to everything that is alive. This pulsation of existence has the quality of expansion and contraction, dying and renewal. Each microcosmic cycle within our cells is reflected in the macrocosm in the galaxy, in one incredible, interwoven, interdependent system. For a moment, think about the rhythms and cycles that are part of our body's functions. We have already spoken about the breathing cycle, the moment to moment breathing wave of inhalation and exhalation that exchanges oxygen and energy through our bodies, and our heartbeat that in turn facilitates the delivery of oxygen to every cell in the body. Now, take the simple example of the relationship between a tree and the respiratory tract. Our respiratory mechanism from the trachea down to the alveoli (air sacs) looks very much like an upside down tree. Trees are nature's lungs! And as we breathe in oxygen and breathe out carbon dioxide, trees breathe in carbon dioxide and breathe out oxygen. This is a great example of the perfect and harmonious relationship that we have with all of nature.

Now consider the circadian rhythm that regulates our sleep and wake cycle that is so intricately linked to the sun, as we've seen. Think about the cycles of the moon in relation to the menstrual cycle. It is no coincidence that the average menstrual cycle is 28 days, corresponding to the 28-day lunar cycle. In ancient times, when women lived close to the earth, their menstrual cycles correlated closely to the cycles of the moon. During my days at the hospital, I remember noticing that on the nights of the full moon, we saw more cases of gunshot wounds and cases of assault coming through the doors of the trauma unit. The moon was clearly having an effect on the psyches of people. The power of nature was making itself felt.

And how can we forget the most powerful example of nature's cycles – the seasons – a cycle that we can't help but be aware of and be affected by, even if we are living in the city. What we probably are not aware of, however, is how affected we really are. We got a sense of this with Leo's story in chapter 3, when we touched on eating with the seasons. The seasons affect our mood and energy state more than we realise. For example, the end of winter is always the most challenging time for Isabella. Her eyes and skin feel dry, and she is more prone to anxiety. According to Ayurveda, she has a Vata (Wind) body type, which has a dry and cold quality. Living in harmony with the seasons and her body would mean adapting her internal and external environment accordingly. Practically, this may entail having a humidifier at her desk and in her bedroom, and eating foods that are high in natural oils.

Of course our own authentic energy will get depleted if we disconnect with this system we are a part of. But how does a busy stressed person living in a built-up city environment practically ensure an adequate dosage of nature to support optimum energy and health? As we've been emphasising throughout this book, the first step is to create an awareness to reflect on the current role of nature in our lives. Don't forget that our own body is a natural environment. Therefore, just turning our attention to the source of energy that resides in the body and the breath qualifies as a recovery loop.

Spend time in your garden: If you are fortunate enough to have a garden, then spend time in it daily. It is a simple and easy way to establish a greater connection with it. It may be something that you already do, but perhaps you could be more aware of nature's activities in your garden through the season. If you don't have a garden, get some pot plants for your patio or balcony, learn about them and make an effort to nurture them.

Green up: Transform your home and work environment into a living space with plants that energise and oxygenate your environment.

Soak up the rays: Find a way to absorb 20 minutes of morning or afternoon sunshine daily. I'm not advocating sun tanning and dangerous exposure to the sun; the skin cancer scare has sadly resulted in the creation of a negative perception of sun exposure and, as a result, most of us living in cities and working

Guideline for activating recovery loops throughout the year
Daily: At the beginning and end of every day, with micro recovery loops throughout the day
Weekly: Half a day
Monthly: A full day
Quarterly: A whole weekend or long weekend.

in offices are experiencing the negative effects of inadequate exposure to the sun through low vitamin D levels and a subsequent disruption of the endocrine system.

Nature booster: Give yourself a booster dose of nature on weekends. Find a spot of nature close to home where you can breathe and absorb the energy of running water, trees or mountains.

Get out of the city: Take yourself out of the city at least every three months for a weekend or long weekend where you can go for long walks, swim in the sea or look up at the night sky.

Walk barefoot on the grass: This is known as 'earthing'. This is an effective way to tap directly into the earth's electromagnetic field. It balances the endocrine system and soothes the nervous system. It has even been shown to have an effect on red blood cells, making them less sticky, thereby reducing the risk of cardiovascular disease.

> Energy Formula
> *Nature-based recovery loops daily, weekly, monthly and quarterly = authentic energy*

Mind Intelligence

CHAPTER 9

The effect of technology

While we all have the same primal stress response, our perception of what is stressful is different for each of us based on our past experiences.

> **NEO'S STORY: THE NEW MILLENNIUM MALADY**
> **Name:** Neo Khubeka
> **Age:** 26
> **Character traits:** Authenticity, being a people pleaser
> **Life-changing experiences:** Parent's divorce
> **Stress catalysts in last two years:** Pressure of being an entrepreneur
> **Stress indicators:** Skipping meals and living on coffee, neck stiffness
> **Presentation on energy zone map:** Danger zone

The scene was perfect. Just as she had planned it. The hazy dawn sky was the perfect backdrop. The rising sun teased the cool morning air. The hiss of gas and fire sliced through the silence as the hot air balloons floated up towards the sky. The tour group that she had planned this event for was mesmerised.

Meantime, back on the ground, as Neo captured the image on her iPhone and loaded it on to Instagram, she lost the moment. A WhatsApp notification popped up from her sister with the picture of her new puppy, and three more emails appeared from the last time she refreshed her inbox 10 minutes ago. An email from a media liaison person requesting an interview for a magazine, another from a travel agent who was unable to come through for an event. There was one email from her graphic designer with a complaint that she hadn't been paid on time. Neo flitted from one emotion to the next, without even knowing it: puppy-induced warmth and fuzziness moved to irritation and then quickly to guilt for the late payment. But to Neo, it all felt the same. Almost every experience tightened the knot in her belly and fuelled her pounding heart. A feeling that had become normal.

She responded to all three emails, typed a quick message back to her sister with some cute heart emoticons and logged onto her internet banking site to do the payment. By the time she looked up from her phone, the balloons had shrunk and were almost out of sight.

She tightened up even more inside. She had hoped to get more pictures for the blog. She would have done anything for a cup of coffee but there was none in sight. She lit up a cigarette instead. It was the first time that Neo had to start the day this early since her days at 'The Firm'. That felt like a lifetime ago. In many ways it was.

Neo is part of the Net Generation: born in the nineties, smart, adaptable and urgently seeking meaning, pleasure and success. She graduated from university and emerged into the working world with hope, confidence and a law degree in hand. Her path was clearly mapped. She would finish her articles and get into litigation, just as her father had. But three years post articles, she realised that her rise up the career ladder was becoming inversely proportional to her happiness. She felt trapped within protocols and systems. Law restricted her creative mind to formulae and precedents. She craved free expression of words, thoughts and ideas. Her only creative outlet was through her wardrobe, and when she started defaulting to wearing mostly black, she knew that something needed to change. At the age of 24, Neo experienced a full blown crisis of meaning. She blogged about it, drawing on the stories of others who had quit their corporate career to follow their passion and become entrepreneurs. On weekends, she visited markets, joined an art class, went on hikes, signed up for meditation workshops and planned fun weekend trips out of the city. She began to mingle with the hipster crowd and felt like she belonged. She was unashamedly vocal about all her experiences, dreams, hopes and fears.

Her blog began to grow in popularity and soon she was getting over 2000 hits per day. Her readers were drawn to her authentic writing style and ability to stretch herself out of her comfort zone beyond the confines and restrictions of her legal career. Businesses began to approach her to write about them. She was even getting paid advertising on her blog. As time went on, Neo began to feel torn and divided between the two very separate worlds that she had created. She could feel her energy levels plummet on a Sunday evening as she anticipated the week ahead at the office. On weekends she came alive and her eyes sparkled. Neo became increasingly frustrated by her situation and wanted to live her passion for creativity through her work. Fear created the conflict, fear of the unknown, fear of the loss of a steady income.

One morning she woke up and knew it was the right time. At the age of 26, Neo quit her legal career and became an entrepreneur. Her blog had opened the path to a more creative and unconventional career path. She called her business 'SoulScape', an events company that crafted meaningful and soulful experiences for couples, families and business teams.

Her business and legal mind was a great help. Neo was in her element. She met the most interesting and eclectic people, got to experience wonderful, new, undiscovered parts of the city and country. She was high on a creative buzz. She stayed up at night thinking about new places to visit and unique ways to craft soulful and memorable experiences. Within a year, Neo's business had grown to a point where she needed to employ someone, but couldn't quite afford it. Besides, the thought of handing over work to someone else terrified her. She needed to be involved to ensure that no detail was lost.

On the social media platform, Neo had become a trendsetter and influential voice in the world of creative entrepreneurship. She had over 5000 followers on Facebook, 7500 on Twitter and Instagram, and her blog was well known. Aspiring entrepreneurs constantly sought advice and inspiration from her. Her nature was to help and always oblige. Neo inherited her warmth and compassionate nature from her mother who never said 'no', and always put the needs of others before her own, not wanting to disappoint anyone.

I met Neo on a weekend retreat we were running on energy management. She thought it would be a good service offering for her clients but wanted to experience it for herself first. She arrived 25 minutes late because she had missed two turnoffs on the highway. She lost focus while on the phone to a new client and didn't hear Google map's directions. And her battery was dying. By the time she arrived, she was frazzled and embarrassed. Punctuality was important to her.

Neo integrated into the group quickly. She was warm, open and likeable. Part of the discussion in the workshop was the impact of technology on our energy. It was funny to observe that even while having that conversation, she stole glances at her cellphone, which remained firmly at her side throughout the day, and even though her phone was turned on silent and was face down, every few minutes, she would habitually check to see if she had missed a message.

When we went through the energy zone map, Neo ticked almost all the behavioural symptoms in the danger zone and even some of the physical ones. She was wired all the time. She felt as if her mind was on a racecourse and that the race was not coming to an end. She woke up frequently in the middle of the night to check her phone and even answered emails at that time. It gave her some degree of comfort that she had dealt with it and it would reduce her morning 'to do' list. When planning an event, she covered every possible scenario in her mind. She had Plan A and 20 contingency plans to cover every possible eventuality. When doing research for a job, she jumped from one website to another, skimming through articles and often losing focus on what she had originally set out to do. She found it difficult to lock her attention down to just one thing and felt that even though she was busier than ever, she was achieving less in any given amount of time. Her work crept into her social life and her phone became a third wheel in her relatively new relationship. She found it difficult to relax, focus on a book or even watch a movie without her attention being scattered in a hundred different places. Her conversations were constantly interrupted by pings and message alerts. Physically, her system was taking strain from the effects of constant high levels of adrenaline. Her shoulders were hard as rocks and she was constantly at the chiropractor having her spine adjusted.

The energy retreat was a big wake up call for Neo. She realised that she was entangled 'in the web', and it was extracting all the juice and passion with which she initially started her business. Once again, Neo saw a hard truth. She was unhappy, wired (literally and figuratively), and exhausted.

Even from our initial interaction at the retreat, I could see that Neo was part of a growing and worrying global phenomenon of the new millennium. She was experiencing digital burnout or 'technostress'. She had become a slave to the device and a system that initially supported her life and work was now beginning to drain it. Google, one of the leaders of the digital age, has identified this phenomenon, and together with top neuroscientists and mindfulness experts have initiated an entire mindfulness-based programme called 'Search Inside Yourself' to support focus and productivity. We are in an age where it is impossible to keep up with information overload as more and more communication happens digitally and occurs via social media. While technology is advancing at lightning speed there is concern about the impact of technology on our health, minds and relationships. Behavioural scientists are examining the nature of our addiction to our devices and neuroscientists are studying the effects of a digitised life on our brains. Texting and driving is becoming as big a problem as drinking and driving. In some cities in China there are even dedicated texting and walking lanes. While we can put external measures in place, some internal mechanisms are required more urgently.

Neo recognised that she needed to implement some strategies to take back control of her life and energy. She never really considered the connection between her health and energy levels and her relationship with technology. She hadn't even considered her relationship with technology up to that point.

Technology and mindfulness

Throughout this book, we have referred to our built-in energy-giving mechanism of the reactive fight–flight response and the need for recuperation through the 'rest and recover' mode. We have emphasised that this mechanism is unable to keep up with the intensity of our technology-based life and is causing havoc on our energy system.

The fact that the brain is plastic and adaptable to our experiences has been a relatively recent discovery in neuroscience and the implications are worrying. While the brain has adapted to split attention and instant gratification, as well as always being on, the body is suffering the effects. The body is unable to keep up and technostress is becoming a very real problem.

Studies have shown that every time we open an email, a surge of cortisol floods the system. Dopamine, the hormone that is released when we are rewarded, is released when we receive a text message from a social contact. It makes sense that checking our phone compulsively becomes an addiction and that we experience disconnectivity anxiety. The constant deluge of information from emails, instant messages, Twitter, Facebook and Instagram means that the focus of the conscious mind (see chapter 10 for an explanation of subconscious processing and the conscious mind) is constantly being tugged and split, and in the process being drained of its resources. While it is wonderful that we have access to so much information so quickly, emails add to our 'to do' list, triggering anxiety; Twitter feeds might infuriate you because of social injustice, a Facebook feed might make you feel inadequate when you see pictures of your friend's holiday on an exotic island. While some of the information that we are exposed to might be neutral, a great deal of what we choose to expose ourselves to has a very real effect on our physiology. Without us being aware of it, our amygdala gets fired in reaction to a large percentage of what we are exposed to and we can easily get stuck in a state of adrenalised energy and reactivity. And that feeling is addictive. The more we have, the more we need. Our cells become more switched on to these stress hormones and we need even more. Before we know it, we have become habitual techno addicts and a slave to our devices.

Technology also has interesting implications for the way we relate to ourselves and others. Behavioural scientists have seen that social media tends to highlight certain behavioural tendencies. For example, Facebook might exacerbate stress in someone with a narcissistic personality trait if not enough people 'liked' their selfie, or if they don't have as many Facebook friends as someone else. Someone prone to depression might spiral down by a negative comment or perceive posts in a negative way. How we are perceived by social media has now become a measure of success. In other words, the digital world tends to highlight personality traits that we may or may not have been aware of.

In Neo's case, her fear of not disappointing others, not always being available and not missing an opportunity meant that she was constantly tuned into her device. She repeated the action of checking her phone and moving from app to app so often that the neurons began to wire together to entrench the neural pathways so that the unconscious habitual behaviour prevailed. What she believed to be multitasking was simply rapid switching from one task to another. We now know from neuroscience research that it is in fact impossible to multitask. The conscious mind is only able to focus on one task at a time. Every time we task switch and shift our attention from one thing to another within seconds, we are drawing on our precious mental energy resources. Having a conversation on the phone while checking emails might seem like a time saver, but in fact it's an energy drainer and the quality of each action ultimately gets compromised.

Neo committed to shifting the power dynamic with technology and put herself in charge again. But before she could do that, I suggested that she simply become more mindful of her current relationship with her digital devices. What unconscious habits had she developed? How often did she check her phone? How much time was she spending in front of her computer or iPad? How much of that time was actually productive?

She noticed that when she sat down to do a piece of writing or research, she would get distracted by an email notification that would pop up or a WhatsApp message that she answered immediately. By the time she returned to her original task it would be ten or sometimes 20 minutes later – and by that time she had lost her train of thought. She was embarrassed to admit that many times her cellphone even accompanied her to the bathroom where she would attend to emails. That week she spent most of her lunch date with her best friend on a call to her potential client. Her relationship with her phone was really an expression of her relationship with the world. There was a real awareness of her need to please and always be available. She had very few boundaries. That very week, Neo celebrated her birthday and was treated to a decadent dinner by her boyfriend. In that time, he had answered three calls. She felt disrespected and angry. She realised that her friend had probably felt the same just a day earlier.

Neo began to implement strategies so that technology would support rather than drain her energy. She decided that she would divide her 'digitised' time into three parts. The first part was purely work related. The second was inspiration time. This was time to browse the internet, listen to a TedX talk, play around on Pinterest and download music. The third chunk was social time to catch up with friends and reply to personal mails.

As challenging as it was, Neo started to practise 'mindful connection'. She trained herself to stay focused on one task at a time until it was completed. In this way, she found that she completed more tasks in one day rather than having many balls in the air at the same time, which greatly reduced her anxiety. What she found to be most helpful was taking a breath after every email, phone call, meeting or task, as a way to 'wrap it up' and recoup her energy before moving on to the next thing. The insertion of the 'micro' recovery loops made a big difference to her state of mind and she began to feel more in control again.

She made a concerted effort to keep her phone out of sight whenever she was in the company of someone, whether it was a friend, colleague or client. She took inspiration from the words of someone who met Nelson Mandela and reflected that whenever Madiba met someone – even if it was for a brief second – he made them feel as if they were the only person in the room. She aspired to relate to others in that way.

Just making a few of these changes, Neo felt the quality of her life improving. In no way did she feel that she had perfected the skill; it was a constant work-in-progress, but at least she felt like she wasn't skimming the surface of life anymore. By being more present, she was able to notice more, and experience life more fully. She felt like she was living deeply and widely at the same time.

Of all the factors in our lives that impact on our energy, I worry about technostress the most. As technology is advancing at a blinding speed, we are exposed to more information than we have ever been in the history of humanity. Neural pathways in the brain are firing in ways they never have and our brains are constantly being shaped in response to the information and how we process it. However, statistics are revealing that the 'energy crisis' that we are facing is a warning that we are not keeping up. Susan Greenfield, an Oxford University professor who studies the mind, is worried too. She says that through our interaction with information technology, we are developing a better IQ and memory, and are able to process information faster, but also warns that rather than being the slaves of technology, we should be harnessing it in ways that support our energy and growth. We have a responsibility to ourselves and future generations to go back to basics so that we don't strangle and suffocate in the digital web and lose our vitality and humanity in the process.

Eight ways to mindfully untangle

1. *Just observe*
   Start by noticing how you relate to technology. How much time do you spend on your devices? How much time do you spend away from your devices? What do you use your devices for? What habits have you developed that relate to information technology that could be draining you? Do you habitually check your phone? Do you tend to multitask? Do you find yourself getting distracted when you're working on a task? Does technology invade the time you spend with family and friends? When last did you read a real book? When last did you write with a pen on paper? If you use social media, what is the nature of the feeds you receive? Do those posts mostly drain or support your energy?
2. *One thing at a time*
   Research is clear that excessive multitasking is harmful to the brain of people who are online more than 10 hours a day, having less grey matter than those who spend less than two hours a day online. Decide what you are working on and consciously focus on doing that one thing. If it is a particular task requiring more focus and concentration, limit the possibility for interruption. For example, turn your phone onto silent, and resist the urge to get pulled into answering a message. In most instances it can wait. In his book *i Disorder*, Larry Rosen advises noticing how long you are able to focus on one task before switching to another, and noticing what distracts you. Then redesign your environment to make it more conducive to focus. He also advises taking tech breaks every 15 minutes, even if it means stretching and taking a few deep breaths.

3. *Eye contact*

We have developed the habit of communicating digitally even if someone is sitting right in front of us. Our interactions are so much richer when we have personal contact. We sense and empathise more and pick up on nonverbal cues when we speak to someone directly. Create more opportunities to pick up the phone or walk to someone's desk instead of sending an email or text. Another aspect of digital communication is the reactive, knee-jerk responses to emails and messages without really considering the impact of the words and language. This opens up the possibility for misinterpretation, and assumptions could be avoided if we created 'e-gaps' before answering messages, especially those that have triggered an emotional reaction.

There is another aspect to this on the other spectrum, which tends to overcompensate for the lack of one-on-one contact. The phenomenon of sending meaningless pleasantries back and forth can be a real time and energy drainer. For example:
EH: Ok, lunch confirmed for 1pm
TR: Great, I look forward to seeing you then
EH: Me too
TR: Thank you
EH: Pleasure
TR: Cool
EH: Great
TR: Until later
EH: Fantastic

Three's a crowd! Put your phone away when you're socialising or in a meeting or having a meal. Who are you really with? Close the loop.

As you are working on a task, for example, writing an email, doing research or writing a proposal, activate micro recovery loops after each one of them. Take a breath or two, give yourself a stretch to re-boot your energy before moving on to the next thing. Sometimes we get so pulled into the screen that we don't pay attention to the physical body. We only tend to notice tension in the shoulders or in the back when we feel pain.

4. *Be discerning*

    Be conscious of the information that you allow into your space. How much negativity from media and social media do you allow into your space? And what is the impact on your energy? Be mindful of what you watch and listen to, and how it is benefiting you. Who do you follow on social media and why? Detox your space from the people and information that drain your energy. When it comes to watching television, do you waste time and energy mindlessly flipping channels because you are bored and tired? Choose what you enjoy watching on television and allocate the time to watch just that programme. Having the television in the background fills your awareness with unnecessary clutter. Each of us are unique in the way that our brain works and what supports our focus. For some of us, listening to music while working supports focus, while for others it is a distraction. Be aware of how your brain works to support focus and energy. Psychologists call this 'metacognition', which is the ability to be aware of your own mental processes and understand your brain and how you deal with incoming information.

5. *Daydream*

    Make time to be bored and to daydream. If you are waiting in a queue for transport or a meeting, every now and again, resist the urge to take out your phone and flip through your mails, messages and updates. Use the time to just be aware and notice your surroundings.

6. *Pen it*

    In the digital age, our fingers are a blur across the keyboard. We type and text so much that this neural pathway has become highly developed and almost automatic. We don't write as much anymore so we are forgetting how to! Writing activates a different part of the brain than typing does. It unlocks creativity and strategic thinking, a source of mental energy.

7. *Unplug and tune in*

    Unplugging for a half or a full day acts as a powerful macro recovery loop. Be in nature regularly to restore your energy.

Research has shown that interacting with a natural environment supports a focus that engages all the senses, which allows the overworked parts of our brain to recover. Even a nature break of a few minutes is effective in re-booting the brain. Interestingly, research on the subject has also shown similar benefits when viewing pictures of nature for ten minutes.

8. *Wind-down ritual*

   Another habit of the digital age is taking our devices to bed or falling asleep in front of the television. As we mentioned in our chapter on sleep, the backlight from these devices interferes with the production of the sleep hormone melatonin, which will, in turn, affect the quality of our sleep. Switching off from all electronic devices at least 30 minutes before bedtime will support far better quality of energy restoration.

> Energy Formula
> *Unplugging + one thing at a time + digital discernment*
> *= authentic energy*

CHAPTER 10
Mindful living

Neural pathways in the brain are firing in ways they never have and our brains are constantly being shaped in response to the information and how we process it.

> **MARCUS'S STORY: ANTI-HIJACK**
> **Name:** Marcus Friedman
> **Age:** 44
> **Character traits:** Graciousness; inability to express and communicate feelings
> **Life-changing experiences:** Being abandoned by his father at age 5
> **Stress catalysts in the last two years:** Promotion to CFO
> **Stress indicators:** Lower back pain; use of sleeping pills
> **Presentation on energy zone map:** Danger zone

The pre-dawn air was cool and alive with possibilities; the night sky turned luminous as the sun teased the horizon. Before the world filled up with the noise of tantrums and traffic, Marcus Friedman was soaking up the silence of the morning with his usual five-kilometre run. The monotonous rhythm of his feet hitting the ground in synchrony with his laboured breath unlocked his strategic mind. Beads of sweat surfaced below his recently receding hairline. The road was open. The air was sharply crisp. His mind was clear: problems that plagued him at the office suddenly turned into possibilities.

Marcus had always relied on this solitary time to think, regroup, strategise and deal with particularly perplexing problems. His role as the chief financial officer at an investment bank demanded that his thinking was always laser sharp, and both focused and broad. His journey to the C-suite was a rocky tangent and he still had a lot to prove in the fragile economic state. That day, Marcus failed to find the answers he was looking for. The questions were of a different nature. The feeling of guilt and shame from the previous night's events drowned out all thought of strategies or stock price.

He couldn't quite figure out where it all went wrong. He and his wife had been up most of the previous night with their four-year-old daughter who had a tummy bug. Earlier that morning he had an early morning meeting set up with the COO who arrived 20 minutes late without apology. For Marcus, lack of punctuality reflected disrespect. But once again, Marcus said nothing. Marcus raised the bar for himself and for others at the same level of management, which meant that, for a lot of the time, he walked around heavy with disillusionment. He loathed nothing more than corporate politics. He refused to engage with the drama. That day, Marcus found it harder to keep himself in check. It seemed that it took a great deal of effort and energy to regulate his irritability, but despite this, he managed to retain a calm exterior. Marcus arrived home hungry, irritable and exhausted. He heaved a sigh of relief as he unlocked the front door. His next breath was a yelp that sent him flying across the hallway and landing on his face, as he tripped over his six-year-old's magnificent Lego construction.

His wife, Kathy, had also had a rough day, between doctor's appointments, school runs and seeing some clients at her home-based physiotherapy practice. Dinner was a blurred event that night, as Marcus zoned out. He felt depleted and Kathy's voice became a distant drone. Surely, she could have chosen a better time to discuss a weekend away with the in-laws? Even at the best of times, the mere thought was excruciating – but that day, it just felt like too much to bear. He noticed the mounting tension in his body and felt his jaw clenching. Marcus understood that Kathy was trying to heal her fractured relationship with her brother and was willing to put his feelings for him aside. But that evening there was no energy for compromise and logic. Kathy found his clipped response offensive. She was just trying to do the right thing and would have appreciated more support. The argument seemed to take on a life of its own. Neither Marcus nor Kathy were able to access their usual logic.

As the argument tipped over the edge, Marcus's pupils began to dilate with rage, his cheeks turned crimson, his mouth went dry and his belly churned. It was when Kathy called him a 'selfish swine' that he flipped. Before he knew what was happening, he had Kathy pinned up against the wall and his arm was lifted ready to strike. It was her look of absolute terror and shock that jolted him back to rationality.

Kathy slept in the kids' room that night and Marcus was left with anguished restlessness. Never before had Marcus lashed out at anyone with violence, let alone someone he loved more than breathing itself. He needed to understand why he had reacted out of character and with such outrageous intent. Never before had he felt so out of control. He vowed that this would never happen again. His confusion and shame were the catalyst to his ultimate journey of self-discovery. This is when he called me.

What Marcus had experienced is a common behaviour pattern that we have all experienced in some form. He blew his top. Something about those words triggered him and he acted irrationally. And so had Kathy, by calling him a 'selfish swine'. She certainly didn't mean it. Marcus dived into survival mode and in defence of the 'attack', his knee-jerk reaction in that moment had a negative outcome for both himself and everyone involved. Marcus's logical higher functioning mind had been hijacked by the emotional and instinctive part of his brain. Marcus had experienced what is called an 'amygdala hijack'.

Marcus walked into my consultation room with a stooped posture, his body heavy with shame. As Marcus talked me through the events of the last few days, I began to understand how it had unfolded the way it had. As I took Marcus through what he had experienced in that moment, it helped him to make sense of what had happened and how the stress of the preceding months had a big role to play in his reaction that evening. Through his understanding of the neurophysiology of that experience, he felt far more empowered to deal with what he was feeling.

For Marcus to gain a clearer understanding of his behaviour that night, we needed to go back to the explanation of the brain function and design. I explained to Marcus that the human brain is designed in an ingenious way to process and coordinate billions of functions every second. The brain is organised in three sections, with each part responsible for coordinating a different function. The most ancient part of the brain is the brainstem, housing all the structures that support the body's basic functioning: heart rate, respiration and temperature regulation. This is a rather 'simple' part of the brain, not really required for higher functioning. The limbic or emotional brain processes the more complex functions of memory and emotion. It also coordinates signals coming into the sensory system and to our body.

A particularly interesting structure of the limbic brain is the 'hippocampus', which serves as the brain's memory bank. All our experiences get imprinted here, whether this memory is conscious or unconscious. The hippocampus has a direct connection to a little almond-shaped structure called the amygdala which triggers the survival based fight–flight response of which we've been speaking. The amygdala will fire up the signal in response to instinctive threats, but also any perceived threat. What is perceived as a threat depends on the memories that are stored in the hippocampus. While we all have the same primal stress response, like reacting to a loud bang, for example, our perception of what is stressful is different for each of us based on our past experiences.

The most sophisticated and complex part of the human neurological system is the neocortex, the 'new' brain, which is a highly developed system of neural networks organised in four lobes on each side of the brain, each one having a different function. The occipital lobe at the back of the skull interprets visual input, the parietal lobe processes other sensory stimulus, while the temporal lobes, situated above the ears, are responsible for auditory perception and understanding meaningful speech. The frontal lobes are of particular relevance to this conversation, being home to the centre of conscious awareness, attention, focus and rationality. Of interest to us in terms of understanding energy is the left prefrontal cortex, the most 'human' part of the brain or what I see as the 'heart brain'. It can also be seen as the C-suite of the brain, where all the executive functioning and decision-making happens. While this is an oversimplification of the anatomy of the brain, it is the foundation of our understanding of the two fundamental operating systems of the brain, the subconscious and conscious mind.

Ninety-five per cent of the brain's functioning is subconscious. In order to conserve energy for the billions of functions that the brain has to regulate, it has evolved to process information at a rate of twenty million bits of information every second! This means that all our habitual thoughts, actions, habits and patterns that are set in cell memory and muscle memory, get transferred across to the subconscious mind as an energy-saving mechanism, freeing up space for the conscious mind to focus on learning new information, making decisions and paying attention and staying focused. The conscious mind housed in the neocortex processes information at a far slower rate of 40 bits of information per second.

In Daniel Kahneman's book *Thinking Fast and Slow* he refers to the subconscious processing as 'system 1' and the conscious mind as 'system 2'. To illustrate how system 1 and 2 operate in harmony, consider the following example of driving a car on a route that you travel every day, say from home to work. Initially, when the route was still unfamiliar, you needed your conscious mind to pay attention to where you were going, but as the route became more familiar, and practised, the neural pathways became hardwired and the action of driving switches across to system

1, to free up energy for system 2. The conscious mind, and its processing unit in the cortex, works most efficiently when it works in spurts and sprints, and needs to be supported by a rich supply of glucose and oxygen. It needs recovery time and replenishment of its energy resources. Modern life, time pressure and technology have demanded more from our conscious mind. System 2 has not been designed to multitask and work at the pace that is demanded from modern life. As a result, we default to system 1 reactive behaviour. We switch to autopilot mode and default survival-based programming to operate our daily lives.

Constant decision-making, dealing with multiple demands in the working day and putting effort into 'keeping our cool' leaves less energy for the more rational 'system' to take over. This also occurs when we are constantly internalising our emotional reactions, in an attempt to display a calm exterior demeanour. What is happening chemically and emotionally on the inside is a bubbling smouldering cauldron that explodes with the slightest provocation. The more depleted system 2 gets, the more likely we are to default to old habitual patterns of thought, feeling and behaviour that reside in the subconscious mind or system 1. Our willpower is weakened, leaving our rational mind susceptible to 'hijacking' by the survival or fear-based amygdala. In other words we have a severe reaction or emotional outburst that is out of context to the situation. The reactive behaviour is often out of character, leaving us feeling guilty or ashamed once the rational mind has kicked in.

Amygdala hijacks can happen in devastating ways, leaving mass destruction in their wake. Think of severe forms of road rage where people are killed in a fit of irrational anger. More often we experience mini amygdala hijacks in less severe forms, a temper outburst with our kids after a stressful day, a screaming match with a colleague that we regret seconds later.

Amygdala hijacks happen when we are out of resources, mentally exhausted, and disconnected emotionally. It occurs when we have maladaptive coping strategies.

The good news, as I explained to Marcus, is that we have the ability to change our brain through certain practices that focus on slowing down, being aware of our internal state and being more responsive to situations we encounter rather than reactive. Rather than habitually reacting mindlessly to situations, we can develop mindful recognition and train the mind to respond more appropriately.

It is only in the last 15 to 20 years that we have discovered that the shape of our brain is not cast in stone. In fact, it is pliable, plastic and highly responsive to new thought and behaviour patterns. When we activate an action, the neurons that are responsible for making that action or behaviour possible begin to wire together. The more a behaviour is practised, the more the nerves wire together, creating a new neural network or pattern.

When we practise 'being aware of what is happening as it is happening', the prefrontal cortex, the part of the brain that is responsible for attention and focus, lights up. The more this is practised, the more the grey matter in this part of the brain is built up. Research has demonstrated that there is a 30% thickening in the grey matter in the prefrontal cortex of people who practise just 12 minutes of mindfulness a day.

Mindfulness is like gym for the brain. Just like we go to the gym to train and condition our body to be fit, we can apply mindfulness techniques daily in order to live more mindfully.

In that way, self-awareness, empathy, better listening, and rational and creative thinking are reflections of being more 'Mindfit'. We can start building on our body's intelligence and harnessing our mental energy. When we do this, we can retrain the amygdala to fire in the appropriate circumstances and situations. The amygdala can be used for the function it was designed for: to activate energy in true high-demand situations, and can stand back when rationality is required.

Marcus understood the logic but the word 'mindfulness' still conjured up images of meditating monks. He felt far from a meditating monk. However, Marcus's interest was piqued. I explained to Marcus that mindfulness is simply a way of living that is open, attentive and responsive, rather than reactive. It is a way of being that is conscious, adaptable and, at the same time, living in alignment with your values.

The formal definition is 'complete attention on the present moment without judgement'.

Marcus's response was understandable. 'This definition seems vague and impractical. How does this translate into action when you are dealing with a life that feels like a warzone with missiles flying at you in all directions? Discernment, judgement and critical thinking are aspects of thought that are necessary and important, especially in my job,' he said.

I explained that this was even more reason to practise mindfulness. We all develop certain ways to deal with the stressors of life and the human body–mind is designed so that we have the ability to adapt moment by moment to what we are experiencing. However, if we don't involve system 2 in the process, we easily find unconscious ways to cope. We work even harder, fill our lives with even more busyness, we numb ourselves with chemicals and we use food to push our feelings away. In the process, we fuel the stress response even more, we're locked into adrenalised energy and the amygdala gets overstimulated and begins to work against our survival rather than supporting our growth.

This made sense to Marcus and he was ready to take the first step. I told him that he already had. Marcus had a very well-developed system 1, but it was also being overused. It was out of resources because of the constant decision-making, strategising and keeping himself emotionally in check. He did not make enough time for recovery through reflection, downtime and recovery loops. He didn't allow himself an outlet and system 1 took over with devastating consequences.

Marcus's homework was to practise some formal and informal mindfulness exercises and report back to me in two weeks. The first practice was to find ten minutes in his day, preferably in the morning, to watch his thoughts. All he had to do was sit quietly in a comfortable position and focus on his breathing. Every time a thought popped up all he had to do was observe the thought and redirect his focus on his breath. His second task was simply to notice when he was feeling stressed and what that experience of stress felt like – physically, mentally and emotionally. He didn't have to do anything about it except watch his experience.

The first few days Marcus found the first task extremely challenging. It felt like a waste of time. He questioned what the point of the exercise was and he found it almost impossible to quiet his mind. Random thoughts flooding in, he felt a whirlwind of feelings. His mind felt like a natural disaster zone. He didn't think it was working.

The second task he found slightly easier and definitely more interesting. He became aware of how tight his jaw felt, and noticed that his clenched jaw was what brought attention to his stress. He also noticed that listening to the radio on his way from work fed the tension build up in his system and subsequently made the choice to listen to his favourite music instead of the news. That way he arrived home in a calmer state, and was able to give his wife more attention and energy.

Marcus persevered. He began to really enjoy the sessions and his new found relationship with himself. His biggest challenge was this idea of not judging or analysing what he was becoming aware of. He was solution-driven and found it hard to adapt to this idea of observing without doing anything about it. It felt like a cop out. He was developing self-awareness but found himself constantly analysing what he was noticing. This created even more anxiety. He judged his thoughts and behaviour as 'stupid', and 'unnecessary', and his anger started becoming self-directed.

We are creatures of habitual judgement, everything is categorised into 'good or bad', 'right or wrong'. When we can step back and simply be entertained by what we are becoming aware of, we are shifting from system 1 to system 2 and choices and responses can be made from a more rational and empathetic place.

Marcus was also struggling with this concept of 'clearing his mind'. In fact he found it impossible.

The nature of the mind is to think. It is absolutely natural and normal for the mind to feel busy as we begin to quieten down. But the very act of noticing and gentle direction to the breath is the very thing that embeds the pathways of responsiveness and thickens the grey matter in the prefrontal cortex. In other words, the wandering of the mind is like the extension of a muscle and bringing attention back to the breath is the flexion. Every time we guide the attention back to the breath, we are flexing our mental muscle!

Now he was getting it. In the weeks that followed, Marcus began to practise for ten minutes in the morning and evening. In his morning session, he found that creative ideas popped into his awareness and he enjoyed the evening session as a way to wind down. He was also becoming more in tune with his breathing and found that the tension released as soon as he became aware of his breath.

Kathy couldn't believe the change in Marcus. He seemed more present with her and the kids and less distracted. He still found his work environment frustrating at times, but was able to breathe through it. His thinking felt clearer and he enjoyed being more focused. He found that his listening capacity in meetings had improved and that he was able to gather his mental energy and direct it to the task at hand instead of feeling like his attention was scattered. Most of all, Marcus felt happier than he had in a long time. He had come back home to himself.

About mindfulness

Mindfulness has its roots in Buddhism as a contemplative practice that fosters compassion. In recent years, and primarily through the work of Dr Jon Kabat Zinn, this practice was been secularised and systemised into a programme called Mindfulness-Based Stress Reduction or MBSR, which has become widely applied across the globe as a method for managing stress, pain and trauma. Business schools are teaching the method and organisations are integrating it into their wellness programmes. Medical students are being trained to use it with their patients. Mindfulness has become a tool of resilience and a pillar for emotional wellbeing.

In the face of rapid change, uncertainty and technological

advances, the only way we are able to ride the waves of change and grow through it – instead of being drowned by the tidal wave of change – is to find an anchor that can only be found within ourselves. Mindfulness is a way that we can begin to navigate that path inward and live more open heartedly.

It is about relationality, in other words, how we are in relationship to everything, including our thoughts and emotions, minds and bodies; how we can learn to live every aspect of our lives with integrity and wisdom. Many scientific streams, from genomics to epigenetics and neuroscience, are revealing indisputable ways that this relationality has a significant and meaningful impact on every aspect of who we are, our genes and chromosomes, cells and tissues, neural networks in our brain, thoughts and emotions, and even on our social networks.

A study done at the University of California shows that our thoughts and emotions, especially stressful thoughts of the past and future, influence the rate at which we age, right down to the level of our telomeres, the protective DNA caps on our chromosomes that shorten as we age. The study showed that telomere shortening is much more rapid under conditions of chronic stress, and how we perceive stress will determine the rate of the shortening.

The Shamatha Project was a three-month comprehensive and ground-breaking study that demonstrated the effects of mindfulness practice. It showed 30% higher levels of the anti-aging enzymes – telomerase – in meditators, greater resilience in the face of stressors, reduced stress reactivity, and greater decreases in cortisol levels.

Ways to start practising mindfulness

Watch the movie of your mind
Choose a time in your day where you will not be disturbed for ten minutes. Sit in a comfortable position with your back supported. Close your eyes and tune in to your breathing without trying to change it. Notice the feeling of the breath in your belly. Lock your

attention on this feeling. Within seconds you will notice thoughts starting to flood into your awareness. This is normal. Simply notice what the thought is and, without indulging it, gently guide yourself back to the feeling of the breath in your belly. You might go into a stream of thought and get lost in a story before you realise you've done so. This is also normal. Just notice the story and bring yourself back to the breath. Remember that the point of this exercise is not to 'empty the mind', it is to practise being the watcher. Like we extend and flex muscles at gym, we are flexing the muscle of the left prefrontal cortex every time the mind wanders off and we bring it back to the focus of your attention. The more you practise this technique, the more you will begin to experience spaces between thought, and the longer the spaces will become. This exercise can be seen as a formal mindfulness practice. As you progress, you can increase the time to 20 minutes.

Mindful moments
Choose a short activity that you do daily to practise being fully present, for example, brushing your teeth or having a shower or walking to your car. Engage all your senses and feel your whole body. When you notice your mind wandering off, engage your senses again. This doesn't require extra time; you are simply being more mindful and present with what you are already doing. When practising this technique, you are immediately breaking out of stress reactivity and activating a recovery loop.

Mindfulness in action
Make a list of your particular triggers for an amygdala hijack. Is it when your highest values are being threatened or questioned? Is it when you are hungry and irritable? Is it when you haven't slept enough and are feeling exhausted? Can you start to notice when you are about to have an amygdala hijack? Start to notice what your body feels like as if you are about to be hijacked. See if you can override the knee-jerk reaction by taking a step back and noticing what you are experiencing in that moment. Notice what starts to change when you start observing and not reacting.

> ### Energy Formula
> *Notice + present moment + non-judgement = authentic energy*

CHAPTER 11

Living in the present

The more aware we are, the more opportunity we have to respond to the situation in a way that will save us more energy.

NASEEM'S STORY: NOWHERE VS NOW HERE
Name: Naseem Sayed
Age: 53
Character traits: Zest for life, stubbornness
Life-changing experiences: Birth of his twin daughters
Stress catalysts in last two years: Being diagnosed with bladder cancer
Stress indicators: Excessive smoking
Presentation on energy zone map: Burnout zone

Aluminium windows framed moving pictures of the outside world. A normal world, with normal people. And trees. And pretty flowers. Seven people sat in soft recliners that didn't belong in a hospital. You could tell those who were familiar with the process. They came prepared. Knitting, books, Sudoku. They wore an expression that spoke of something between resignation and acceptance.

His breath ceased for a second as the needle pierced through his thinning skin. He wasn't sure what he feared more, the cancer or the chemo. The smell of the chemicals haunted him long after the first session. It stuck to everything. It was everywhere, in his nostrils, on his clothing. It came through the pores of his skin, a constant reminder of his borrowed time. Precious time, and now contaminated by constant nausea, deep fatigue and pain. The diagnosis came in stages. Every step on the road was bittersweet. Offering hope. And now, he realised that even hope was relative. For two years he thought that it was an enlarged prostate, something that came with age, or at least, that is what he was told. But the pain in his back just got progressively more intense, pulling his attention into his body. Naseem had spent almost half of the year in between airports, but even first-class luxury did nothing to soothe his discomfort. He had never felt the impact of jet lag before. He had immense capacity for work. All his energy got poured into planning, negotiating and crafting strategies. He was a sought-after strategy consultant for some of the biggest companies and governments across the globe. In the previous year, the pain and discomfort he felt forced him to stretch out his projects and focus on more local work.

The diagnosis of bladder cancer was a shock and a strange relief. Now he knew for sure what was causing the constant, nagging pain. There was no need to speculate anymore. He didn't do well with not knowing. But before he even allowed himself to feel the impact, he did what came naturally. He created a plan of action. He gathered a team of the best doctors and went with what they suggested. He was sure that within the next year life would feel normal. But now normal took on a whole new meaning. They said that the cancer had penetrated the bladder too deeply. It was too far gone. The bladder had to go and, with that, a whole layer of identity. Just as he was settling into the new normal of life without a bladder, the next diagnosis came. Stage 4 cancer. It had spread to his liver, lungs and lymph nodes. Six months was all he had and that was being optimistic.

This was the second round of chemo. Palliative was the word they used. Just buying time. Buying moments. Suddenly moments took on a whole new meaning.

'Oh there you are, old chap.' The familiar voice brought a wave of warmth to his frozen bones. Naseem's best friend Sebastian pushed the swing door open, carrying a portable chess board under his arm. Sebastian's smile pierced through the pain of seeing Naseem in the leather chair looking frail and gaunt. Naseem mirrored it back. It felt so good to see his dear friend again. If anything got him through the chemo sessions, it was the chess sessions with Sebastian. More than that, it was the real conversations.

Sebastian knew loss. It had knocked at his door many times. But he also knew joy and love. Loss had always walked through this door hand in hand with it. Naseem was feeling reflective that day. Over time, the plans faded and strategies crumbled as the future and the present began to merge.

Between the moving of knights and pawns, Sebastian and Naseem chuckled and cried over moments they had shared over the years. Before the 'diagnosis' they had hardly seen each other, both had been caught in their own web of life. In that moment, none of that made sense to Naseem. He hadn't prioritised time for someone he cared about. He felt the physical pain of that.

Naseem tried to play back the movie of his life in the last few years, trying to extract and clutch onto moments that stood out, moments that mattered. The birth of his twins was the last event that made him stop in his tracks. It was the last time he felt so fully present, so completely alive. After that, between nappy changes, feeds and flights, the days moved so fast that the picture felt blurred. It moved too fast. There was nothing to clutch on to. Naseem remembered a time when it was so different.

Naseem grew up in a small town in KwaZulu-Natal. As a child he was intense, contemplative and imaginative. He played in the field, climbed trees, got lost watching the stars in the night sky. He had a particular love for music. Often he got pulled into moments that became a music video in his mind. The leaves would dance to the rhythm of the tune he was listening to, or the neighbour mowing the lawn would be moving in perfect harmony to the song on the radio. In fact, as a child, Naseem believed without a doubt that he had the magical ability to make things move to music. And there in that moment, in the chemo chair, it happened again. Sebastian held the Bishop between his index finger and thumb lightly and deliberately drew it above the chessboard in tune to Beethoven's piano concerto playing in the background. Naseem's music videos were back.

Naseem was a master thinker. He listened attentively, probed deeply and thrived on complexity. He was an instigator, a revolutionary, a maverick who cajoled people from their comfort zone of outdated ideas and thinking, whether it was a CEO or head of state. Naseem pulled no punches; he was forthright in his opinions and stood by them with firm conviction.

He had always relied on his thinking mind to sift logic from confusion and reason from emotion. That's how he moved through the world. If something was painful, upsetting or unnerving, Naseem's default was to go directly to the place he could trust. His mind, his logic. He had the ability to see the clear lines between cause and effect. The more the world demanded of his time and energy, the more energy he spent thinking. The more impact he made on the world, the more complacent he became about the aspects of his life that felt safe and that he could rely on. His body had never failed him, despite the disregard of its basic needs. His relationship was stable and his wife created a structure that facilitated his lifestyle. His children loved him unconditionally and seemed to adapt to his sporadic presence.

So when Naseem, master thinker and strategist, reflected back on his life and little stood out as meaningful memories in the last few years, he began to ask himself some hard questions. Had he aligned his attention to what was most important to him? What would his children remember about him when he was gone? Had he really considered the fact that his attention had a quality to it? Had he really used his mind in the most effective way? What had he done or not done to contribute to his illness? Was it possible to use the power of his mind to reverse his cancer? His questions became existential and penetrated the place where logic resides.

Something opened up in Naseem's awareness in the moment that the music video returned. The answer suddenly became clear to him. It occurred to him that life is nothing but a string of moments. When we pause and reflect on our lives, it is the quality of each of those moments that matter. That is what ultimately determines the quality of our life. And it's the depth of awareness and depth of our presence that will determine how much energy we are able to extract from each moment.

When we are running around doing as much as we can in the shortest amount of time, we bear the risk of skimming the surface of things. We move quickly from one thing to the next, preoccupied and absent to where we actually are, what we are doing and how we are feeling. We walk half alive through a two-dimensional world, losing energy in analysing and worrying, ruminating and judging, suffocated by thought.

As Naseem locked down the checkmate, he pledged to attend to each remaining moment of his life, fully and completely. Even if he was sitting in the chemo chair, with chemicals setting his veins on fire, he'd be right there. Open. Awake. Alive.

I met Naseem just before he was diagnosed with cancer. He found the holistic approach refreshing, fascinated by the possible interconnectedness of what he was feeling physically, mentally and emotionally. It seemed logical to him. When the diagnosis of cancer was made, Naseem clutched onto the holistic perspective as a valuable addition to his treatment, if not the solution for a cure. At that point, Naseem held on to any possibility, a scientifically validated miracle.

Sadly, it didn't work out that way. When his urologist revealed that the cancer had spread, Naseem's dreams and hopes fell away. As Naseem's doctor, or 'healer' as he saw me, I had to make peace with the fact that the healing wasn't about curing, but was more about supporting Naseem to open up to the life he had, completely and fully – whatever that meant.

Despite the pain, nausea and discomfort, Naseem's life took on a magical quality. In the last few weeks of his life, he sat captivated as his son read to him. His heart burst wide open watching his daughter sleep. Water had never been as quenching. The sun rays seeped into every bone. A warm bath soothed his soul. The smell of the summer storm had never made him feel more alive. Something beautiful happened for me too during this time. I began to see life through the eyes of a dying man. And the view was crystal-clear as thinking gave way to awareness. And awareness made space for acceptance, insight and gratitude.

When I attended Naseem's memorial service, I knew for sure that he had succeeded in coming alive as he prepared for death. His friends and family spoke of a man that lived widely, curiously and passionately. They celebrated a man that had learned to live more deeply, who gave all of himself to every experience and every moment that he had. He had 'romanced the ordinary', and had left each person with their own beautiful music video.

The value of living in the present

Living in the present might seem like a simple concept, a clichéd or somewhat vague one. We might understand its value theoretically, but what does it really mean for us, and what does it have to do with energy?

Being present means being fully aware and engaged physically, emotionally and mentally with our current experience. This requires an ability to create a gap between ourselves and our experience, as if we are watching a movie of our lives rather than being part of the movie. This does not mean being passive or complacent. Creating this gap allows an opportunity for us to respond to what we are experiencing, rather than reacting from a habitual place that is running an outdated software program written by our past experience.

Imagine that for ten minutes you verbalised every thought you had in your mind, recorded it and played it back to yourself. What do you think you would hear? Probably jumbled, incoherent, jagged thoughts that flitted from one thing to another. It would be quite amusing and definitely disturbing. You would be forgiven for thinking that you've gone off the rails. The dialogue would be scattered, erratic and cluttered with questions, assumptions and judgements. We would be playing out different scenarios and memories, the dialogue of your mind for just ten minutes.

We know from research that the body does not know the difference between what it is actually experiencing and what the brain is thinking about. In other words, the body will respond to an actual experience or thought about an experience in exactly the same way. So imagine the flood of chemical reactions occurring in our system every time we ruminate on something that has happened in the past or worry about and play out all the possible scenarios that could happen in the future. The stress hormones and neurotransmitters are released in response to these thoughts, which triggers an emotion, further feeding the thought and the physical response.

We constantly leak energy into the past and future as we allow system 1 to run our thinking and fall into the trap of adrenalised energy. The stress/energy response gets activated and has nowhere to go but more deeply into the muscle fibres and cells of our bodies. The jaw tightens, breathing becomes shallower, heart rate increases, the amygdala gets activated and so the cycle goes. The most amazing part is that all this is happening without us even realising it.

The more present we are, the more the body relaxes. The gap provided by present moment awareness is an opportunity for the most appropriate energy response to be activated. The stress energy response can be utilised and activated in real high-demand situations, rather than the imagined ones. The more aware we are, the more we have the opportunity to respond to the situations in a way that will save us more energy.

Being in charge of the quality of our attention allows us to manage our energy more masterfully and to use it in a different way to which we've become addicted. The gap is a creative opportunity for a fresh perspective, an innovative response and productive outcome. The neuroscience of present moment living is compelling and convincing. But more than that, we see the evidence in people who we know live with this quality of awareness.

Dan Brulé, world-renowned expert in the field of conscious breathing and consciousness, spent a year interviewing people who are peak performers in their field, from Stig Severinsen, who holds the world record for holding his breath under water (22 minutes), to top business people. When asked what the common thread in all these individuals was, he said the first common thread was awareness of their breath and the deliberate use of their breath in certain moments. Secondly, they all had a real desire to make a difference in the world, and thirdly, they all had a knack of being able to extract all the juice from life, from all their experiences. While this may sound like an easy thing to do, it is probably the most challenging thing in the world.

Up to now, we have referred to system 1 as the subconscious mind, where all our memories, beliefs, habits and patterns reside. Our habitual behaviours, neural pathways and cells in our body are all part of this system that is designed to free up energy for the thinking mind. When the conscious mind is at work, focusing, concentrating, planning, we are engaging system 2. System 2 requires a great deal of energy; it operates at a slower speed and requires regular replenishment.

The present moment awareness I am referring to in this chapter refers to something a little different. The 'gap' that we create by being the observer of our experience allows us to tap into an energy source that is beyond the operating systems of system 1 and system 2. Let's consider the car analogy.

You are driving a modern car that has a manual and automatic option. The actual car is your physical body. When you put your car into automatic mode, the car practically drives itself. It is easy and requires very little energy. Provided that the car is in good condition and all systems are upgraded and intact, this system works pretty well (system 1). However, when we need more action and more energy or we need to overtake, we shift into manual mode (system 2). But who is driving the car? Who is in control of the steering, the route and the shifting of gears? When we create the gap, we get the sense of who is in control and in charge (who we really are).

The gap allows the bubbling up of energy from its actual source, the natural world. That's why we feel recharged and energised when we are in nature. However, we don't need to make a trip to the mountains to access the natural world. We tend to forget that our bodies are part of the natural world too. Fully engaging our senses wakes us up to our own inner natural world. And we can access it even more deeply through our breath, our ultimate energy source. Through this gap, the creative source bubbles up. An inspired thought, deep insight, an 'Aha' moment and an intuitively felt sense of something, are all experiences of creative energy that uses the conscious mind to process it.

Studies done on the topic of mindfulness and present moment living have clearly demonstrated the link between mind wandering and happiness. In other words, people who live more mindfully are happier. At this point let us remind ourselves that the definition of mindfulness is the awareness of the present moment 'without judgement'. Non-judgement is the key that unlocks the door to the gap.

The more we attend to the quality of our awareness, the more we will have a handle on our energy system. Unlocking the reactive mind is the greatest benefit of mindfulness. When we are able to let things just pass through us without defending, attacking, withdrawing or judging, we can then align our attention and energy on what is most important, and we can use the mind's ability to discern, choose and apply boundaries from a more conscious place that supports, rather than depletes, our energy.

How can we begin to practically apply this way of life?

Develop flexibility of awareness
Play with dimensions of focus. A social gathering or meeting is a good time to practise this, or try it right now as you're reading this. Narrow your focus internally into your body by

focusing on one thing, such as the feeling of your feet on the floor or the breath in your belly. Now broaden your internal awareness to include your whole body. Feel your whole body at the same time. Now shift your attention outside your body and focus on one thing, for example, the words on the page. This is a narrow external focus. Broaden your external focus to include all your surroundings when it is appropriate. Now see if you can experience all the dimensions at once. It is really helpful to be able to play with these dimensions. For example, if we become fixed on a narrow internal focus, like a thought or sensation, we can lose out on information and cues from the outside environment and, conversely, if we are too focused on what is going on externally, we can miss out on vital information that the body is communicating.

Take a breath. Taking deep breaths into your belly and giving a sigh of relief is the easiest and most effective way to pull yourself back to the present moment and release tension that has been stored in the body.

Practise observing
I've been playing with this fun writing exercise of just naming what is, without judging or analysing or qualifying. Grab a note book or a piece of paper. Start writing down everything you observe. For five minutes and without putting your pen down, simply write down what you see, and notice the urge to judge, compare and analyse. For example: wooden door, ticking clock, a stack of books with different shapes, the sound of traffic and birds singing.

Practise deep listening
Otto Scharmer, who created a framework for system transformation called Theory U, identifies four levels of listening.

Level 1: This is when we listen from system 1. What we are hearing has been filtered by our own judgements, opinions, assumptions and belief systems. We hear only what will confirm what we already believe and there is no space for seeing a perspective different from our own.

Level 2: When we move to level 2 listening, we are engaging system 2, the conscious mind. This is also known as factual listening.

Level 3: As we drop deeper into ourselves and listen more with our hearts, we are using level 3 listening. We see through another person's eyes and feel empathy.

Level 4: This level of listening happens through the 'gap' created by being fully present. This is called generative listening. When we listen from here, there is space for new creative ideas to emerge from the space 'beyond mind'.

As we deepen our practice of mindfulness, we are more able to access level 4 listening and generate creative outcomes.

Energy in simplicity

There is an exquisite book written by Sarah Ban Breathnach called *Romancing the Ordinary*. Like Naseem, Sarah woke up to the power of the present moment through her own personal journey and shares her wisdom in this beautiful day-by-day guide. She opens us to the wonder, energy and joy that can be extracted from the simplest and most ordinary things that we take so much for granted until we risk losing something that is important or until we know our time is limited.

Practise romancing the ordinary in your life. Let your senses come alive to the small things, breathing in warm rays of winter sun, the smell of baking bread, the first sip of cappuccino through light milky foam.

> Energy Formula
> *Stillness + open awareness + relaxation = authentic energy*

CHAPTER 12

The neurobiology of change

The trick in creating new energy-supporting habits is getting over the part that is boring, mundane and hard, until it becomes habituated. We have to go through the hard process, the neurobiology of change.

> **JULIE'S STORY: UPGRADING SOFTWARE**
> **Name:** Julie Rheeder
> **Age:** 44
> **Character traits:** Feeling fear and doing it anyway, taking things personally
> **Life-changing experiences:** Trip to India
> **Stress catalysts in last two years:** Starting up her own business
> **Stress indicators:** Binging and purging
> **Presentation on energy zone map:** Danger zone

The thunder clapped. She was jolted out of her computer-induced stupor. That was just before the wave of panic took over. The figures on the spreadsheet were dismal. Julie could no longer deny that her business was in trouble. Without some form of divine intervention she would be forced to consider the possibility of going back to working at the place that she felt had stolen her soul, the prestigious company that for her represented a luxurious prison. She resented the idea of her time being controlled by a boss or system.

Two years previously, Julie Rheeder took a calculated leap of faith and started her own freelance advertising business. She preferred being single. It meant that she could throw herself into work without feeling guilty about sharing her time with a partner or children. It was ludicrous to her friends that she had given up a 40-hour week to work an 80-hour week. Rather that, she told them, than waking up every morning to be a slave to traffic, endless meetings and corporate politics. And besides, being busy kept her out of trouble. She was very aware of how self-destructive she could be when she was bored or had too much time to think. And now, the success of her business had more far-reaching consequences. Her aging parents had just moved into a retirement village and needed her financial support. It was no longer just about her.

After a dramatic two-minute downpour, the rain ceased. The world went quiet. The spreadsheet prevailed. Before panic had a chance to put its hands around her throat, Julie reached for her comfort, her solace, her reliable friend who always managed to take the edge off. Self-judgement seeped through vodka-induced numbness. Maybe she didn't have what it takes to run a successful business. Maybe she should have studied more, gone overseas, stayed in that relationship ...

It was approaching dinner time. The vodka had stimulated her appetite. It was the perfect day for a pizza. A whole one. She deserved it, both the indulgent treat and the disgust she felt from the binging. Then the familiar shame set in. Both the feelings and the food rose up into her chest. She had to get rid of it all.

The pattern of binging and purging first began when she was 15 years old. She remembered the first time she put her fingers down her throat. It was soon after the phone call that her only brother had been killed in a motorcycle crash. They had just had a major argument and a few minutes later, she heard his bike roaring down the road. That was the last time she saw him. The guilt was overpowering, the shame unbearable.

The purging added a strange heightened energy to the mix of shock and grief she felt that day. It made it 'tolerable'. She felt relieved, emptied, in control. A pattern soon started to emerge. She could eat with the family, go out with friends, and no one would notice the purging afterwards. She got to a point when she didn't even have to induce vomiting by sticking her finger down her throat. It became an automatic reaction as soon she bent over the toilet bowl. It started with a meal, and eventually degenerated into anything. It even resulted in her vomiting up water. She had mastered the technique of the 'perfect purge'. There was always a mini high, a release of chemicals that brought relief but which only lasted until the next trigger activated the fear and anxiety all over again. There came a time when Julie could no longer hide it from her family. She saw clinical psychologists and psychiatrists who experimented with various combinations of antidepressants, mood stabilisers and anxiolytics. By the age of 24, she managed to wean herself off most of her medication, except one antidepressant, and got the bulimia under control.

To the rest of the world, Julie was the most capable, courageous, intelligent and kind person. Her friends admired her strength and wisdom, her clients commended her efficiency. But Julie's inner world still felt fractured. In rare moments of calm and peace, she was able to perceive her reality through a clear lens. She knew that the old habit was starting to get out of control again. She understood what triggered her behaviour. Years on the therapy couch had supplied her with enough mental ammunition to psychoanalyse herself to a standstill. Her emotional crutch was becoming a habit. And her habit was becoming an addiction. Only now it was a double addiction. The vodka added another dimension to the old pattern. It took the edge off when the work-induced adrenaline interfered with her sleep. Sometimes it would even help her stay awake. If she was working, she knew just when to throw it all up before the alcohol made her feel woozy. Julie knew something in her life needed to change. And she knew that it had nothing to do with work. She just wasn't ready to admit it to anyone but herself, and even then, it was a fleeting honesty.

Julie cited fatigue as the reason for her consultation with me. She hinted at the anxiety. It was only towards the end of the session that the full story emerged. Her narrative was insightful but had been rehashed to so many doctors and therapists over the years that it felt stale. She knew the lingo and anticipated the usual response.

Julie, like most people who consult with me, wanted her life to feel different, more peaceful, fulfilled, abundant and meaningful. Like most people, she desired change. Logically, she knew what this meant, but felt like there was a gaping black chasm between where she was in her life and what she wanted from it. She wanted fast results with minimum effort. Couldn't I give her something that would cure the anxiety, stop the craving, make her sleep, give her energy, take some weight off?

But on another level, she was asking deeper questions. Why had this old habit crept back after all these years? Why did she feel as if everything was falling apart?

Most of her adult life Julie had been operating in the danger zone, addicted to a feeling of adrenalised energy, subconsciously attracting all the experiences that would feed it. After she got a handle on her bulimia, she found other strategies to manage her inner world. She simply distanced herself from it. She dedicated all her time and energy into working and studying, being the steadfast supporter to her friends and family. Her body was never a comfortable place for her to be, so she put all her energy into a place that did feel controllable – her mind.

Julie was ashamed and disappointed that her old habit had resurfaced. Most of the time, she felt like she had a handle on it, but as soon as she was anxious, sleep deprived and exhausted, for whatever reason, she succumbed to her default comfort, which in turn sparked off a whole cycle of thoughts, feelings and behaviour patterns. Very early on in her life, Julie had subconsciously developed a mechanism to cope with emotional trauma. It was a strategy that may well have been a survival response in that it was triggered by intense and overpowering emotion. These feelings, behaviour and chemical responses had sparked up a specific neural pathway that bypassed system 2, the logical mind. The more the behaviour was practised, the more the neural pathway became entrenched, hardwired and habituated into her subconscious mind.

When I explained habits and addictions in terms of neurobiology and what was actually happening in the brain, Julie felt relief from the self-blame, which had become so familiar, and she felt more empowered to reframe her addictive patterns. However, it was important that Julie was embarking on this process to restore her health and energy, not for anyone but herself. For so much of her life, her choices were governed by external factors and the motivation to change came from a need to please or need to be loved and appreciated. For Julie, to own that her process came from a place of self-respect was a big leap and was the very factor that determined the success of the intervention. It didn't happen immediately. It took a few months and some very dark moments for her to arrive at that point. She returned to my consultation room one day, with a fierce determination in her eyes and soft edges around her mouth. I knew she was there to stay.

As a priority, I needed to help Julie put in the basic pillars for her energy system. While I acknowledged that her relationship with food and her body was layered and complex, we needed to ensure that we were prioritising her body's basic needs, that her sleep was restful and restorative, and that she was eating at regular intervals to maintain stable glucose and neurotransmitter levels. It was very easy for Julie to skip meals and she often did. The days zipped past without her eating a single morsel, and she was unaware that her volatility, reactivity and triggering of addictive patterns were often simply linked to her plummeting glucose levels.

Julie was a natural planner, so I harnessed that ability and got her to plan all her meals for the week ahead and ensure that she went shopping for all the ingredients she needed including fruit and healthy snacks like nuts, rye crackers and hummus, veggie sticks and fruit. This small adjustment proved to make a radical difference while we worked on managing the feeling that triggered her old patterns. I also introduced Julie to the idea of recovery loops to train relaxation and awareness into her system. She was given the simple task of taking regular deep breaths and sighs of relief throughout the day using simple cues like sending an email, ending a call, or stopping at a red traffic light as reminders. I also advised her to begin every morning with a mindfulness practice and end her evening with a wind-down ritual that included a ten-minute breathing practice.

Julie already started to feel calmer and more in charge and thus felt motivated to continue taking more steps towards her wellbeing. The hardest part for Julie was to create a new way of relating to her thoughts and feelings that did not involve self-destructive behaviour. We needed to spark up new neural pathways that would become the foundation of a healthier relationship with herself. Up to that point, she had been unconsciously reacting to her emotions and bypassing the discomfort of feeling her emotions. She distracted herself from her internal world by constantly being busy. And the spaces between work were consumed by taking care of the needs of others. Now she needed to learn to get comfortable with the whole range of feelings and thus respond to them with a new set of behaviours, essentially creating a new habit.

We have explored how habits are the brain's clever way of saving energy. As soon as an action, thought, movement or behaviour pattern is repeated and becomes familiar, it moves across to energy-saving system 1, and the home of habit. The neural pathway becomes hardwired and the pattern automated, freeing up energy for the conscious mind to deal with the tasks that require focus, effort, concentration, attention and learning. Not only mechanical actions like driving are automated, but our thought patterns and feelings can become automated too. For example, the more we feel resentment, envy or guilt, and react to these feelings in the same way, the more we are reinforcing the habit of a feeling and behaviour cycle.

Now this is where this clever system can go wrong. The neurobiological mechanism that was designed to conserve energy is actually sapping energy through the habit of chronically activating the stress response. In other words, the stress response is on autopilot and is running the show without us even knowing it!

Julie needed to become aware of the habits of thought, feeling and behaviour that were becoming destructive, and think about how to reprogramme some new ones. Initially, Julie didn't feel that many of the habits she had developed over the years were all bad. She had a point. Many of her thought and feeling patterns had developed as a way to cope with some really tragic and difficult early life experiences. They were a part of her resilience and her ability to adapt and thrive when she needed to. But now, circumstances had changed. It was not her external environment that was the enemy anymore. She had internalised the enemy. It was living inside her and she was fighting it every day. And the daily battle was leaving her depleted and feeling defeated.

Julie's job was to learn to habituate happiness, energy and joy by unravelling the neural pathways that were taking her in the opposite direction. She had to quickly drop the idea that this was going to be a fast-tracked process if she wanted lasting change. Even though she was already feeling better after just a few sessions, if she stopped, the old pathways would simply take over again. The new pathways were still too fragile. She needed to commit. But that required that she get over the guilt that she was investing all this time and effort in herself. The commitment also required that she stay inspired. Julie soon realised that as she began to go within, she could never be bored by what she discovered about herself. In fact, she was constantly surprised by what she learned and discovered about who she was and what she was capable of. This, more than anything, is what kept her in the process.

In the first few months, it worked for her to embark on my '21 day cleansing programmes' that I designed to cleanse the body and support the creation of new habits. I found that these three-week programmes helped to keep her focused and break certain patterns. She did one for 'no purging', another for 'no alcohol', another three weeks for 'no sugar'. But one day she woke up and asked herself: 'Am I really going to live the rest of my life doing

21-day programmes?' That was the day she realised that she no longer needed to and she acknowledged how far she had come. Looking back at her life after a year, the very idea of purging felt so foreign. She enjoyed a glass of wine on occasion, and was very mindful of her choice to do so. Exercise was part of her daily life and her relationship with food was starting to change. She still had days of feeling weighed down, burdened and worried, but she let them pass and was able to come back to her centre quickly.

Reprogramming our neurobiological patterns

Julie's story is a powerful example of how we have the ability to reprogramme each of our internal software systems that doesn't support energy, meaning and happiness. Beyond all the subconscious programmes that we allow to run our lives is a natural state of calm and peace, our brain can easily adapt and mold itself to reflect new feelings, behaviour and abilities. We are learning through amazing studies in the field of neuroscience and human behaviour about the miraculous abilities of nerve cells to regenerate, wire together and create sophisticated neural connections that reflect our highest human potential. With what science is teaching us about the brain and body now is what mystics have always inherently known. No longer can we afford to have the fatalistic view that we are a product of our genes or past experiences. Through awareness, willingness and practise, we can change our thoughts, habits and biological and hormonal responses to them.

When I made the shift from practising as a regular GP to an integrated doctor with a holistic approach, I began to see clients who were actually more concerned about making changes in their lifestyle rather than just seeking temporary relief. Through the experience of my own life and the lives of the people that I work with, I know that change is one of the hardest things we face as human beings. Change is scary. It requires a great deal of energy, courage and hard work.

I will share with you the typical pattern that I have seen in the change process. I'm sure you will relate and hopefully be encouraged to keep moving, because if you do, change will be inevitable. Authentic energy will be yours. It's science.

Learning a new habit is like learning any new skill. It requires daily practice, consistency and patience. Initially, it demands effort and requires energy. When the brain registers a new experience, new neural connections are created. It feels exhilarating and exciting. But the new skill needs to be practised for the pathway to be entrenched, otherwise it's like fireworks in the sky; it looks and feels wonderful for a second but then it's gone. We constantly crave that same feeling of thrill, exhilaration and new experiences that feed the adrenaline addiction. The more familiar an experience becomes the more boring and dull it feels. That's exactly why diets don't work and why any new programme feels exciting at first, and then fizzles away when it becomes mundane. The trick in creating new energy-supporting habits is getting over the part that is boring, mundane and hard work until it becomes habituated. We have to go through the hard process or the neurobiology of change.

The 7 steps of change

1. *Excuses*: Often the need to change something in our lives doesn't come from a space of inspiration but from the fear of losing something that is most dear to us. For example, when this fear overcomes the fear of change or when our livelihood, a relationship, our families or our very own lives are being threatened by a destructive habit and the shadowy and dark bio-neurological entity that has become entangled in our system. Until we reach that point when the desire hasn't become internalised, we will find ourselves in the place where the intention or desire to change may exist, but we construct the obstacles in the form of excuses. These excuses usually appear as very valid. The most common excuse is that 'there's no time'. Other elaborate excuses will also be found, drawing on

spiritual concepts, a recent article or a past experience. We call on our entire database of information in our minds to craft the excuse that validates and justifies the procrastination, addiction or pattern of behaviour. 'I'll start on Monday', 'It's not the right time', 'I'm just being in the moment', 'I'm listening to my body', 'I need to do X first, before I do Y' are some of the common things we say to ourselves. We stay in a state of 'comfortable misery' and part of us really just wants to stay there.

2. *Blocks*: We may be able to move past step 1 through our own mental effort or from pressure around us and begin to muster up the energy to make some changes, but we come up against some big obstacles that seem to be 'out of our hands'. Life keeps getting in the way – the tyre bursts, we get stuck in traffic, a friend needs our help, there's a crisis at work. A block is just a cleverly disguised excuse that we pin on someone or something else. It seems like 'life's way of preventing the change', and relieves us of the responsibility of making the change.

   This makes sense from a quantum physics perspective where physical objects, thoughts and emotions are merely waves of energy vibrating at different frequencies. Fear and subconscious belief systems resonate at frequencies that will draw the experiences and situations with a similar vibration. In other words, we attract what we fear. Like attracts like, and so the cycle gets perpetuated. This is where many of us halt the process of closing the gap and the old, entrenched neural circuitry takes over as the operating system. Behaviour and body trigger emotions, which feed thoughts, which in turn reinforce the belief systems. The old tired rusty wheel keeps turning.

3. *Awareness*: This is the major crossroads on the path that will determine whether the change will actually be made. At this point, there is an opportunity to create an inward shift that arises from the ownership and acceptance of the old pattern. There is a recognition of the old programming, habits and patterns, and what has given rise to them. There is also a deep acknowledgement of the fear.

At this juncture, as the white flag is raised, an alignment occurs between the desire to change and our most deeply held authentic value systems. The shift is made from being motivated to being inspired. There is a willingness to stand at the top of the cliff and get a bird's eye view of this undiscovered interior territory and ask the questions: What got me here? What is my greatest fear? What will this change really mean? Where does this desire to change come from? What's the alternative? What will I give up or lose as I make this change? What does failure mean? Is this choice in alignment with my most deeply held values?

This is the first choice point. Courage, acceptance, self-compassion and support are required as preparation for the further journey inward.

4. *Taking action*: As we begin to close the gap, we arrive at the point where our intention aligns with our internal state and value system. There is a real and genuine attempt to take the action steps of change. As the new skill set is being learned, neurons begin to spark up different connections and a new neural circuitry is created in the frontal lobe of the brain, the seat of choice and self-awareness. This is usually experienced as quite exhilarating, but sometimes scary as new territory is being discovered. It is easy and natural to want to retreat to what is familiar, and it is important to be vigilant and mindful of how and when the old behaviour shows up. And the old behaviour is guaranteed to creep in as soon as our guard is dropped and we might find ourselves at step 1 or 2 again. 'This is taking too long', 'This is too hard', 'It's not working' is what we will say to ourselves. This is a normal part of the process. Remember that the new pattern has just been fired up but the old circuitry is still deeply entrenched.

The challenge is that the new skill needs to be practised for the new pathway to be entrenched. We constantly crave that same feeling of thrill and exhilaration and new experiences that feeds the adrenaline addiction. The more familiar an experience becomes the more boring and dull it feels. The trick in creating new energy-supporting habits is getting over the part that is boring and mundane until it becomes habituated. Like learning any new skill, it requires daily practice, consistency and patience. Initially, it demands effort and requires energy. We need to constantly affirm the inspired and deep commitment to ourselves and gather the support, encouragement and guidance of those who we trust and who have our best interest at heart, whether that is a friend, coach or mentor.

5. *Crossroads*: All these baby steps on the path of change lead us to another crossroads or major choice point. The new habit has been formed but the old circuits and the old 'self' feels threatened and begins its fight for survival. The new circuitry is being entrenched through the new thoughts, feelings and actions. The cells are no longer receiving their fix of 'feel bad' hormones and will begin to pick fights with the new self. If we engage these battles, the conscious brain and the old subconscious brain will begin a full-scale war. It feels easier at this point to throw in the towel than to continue.

    Be aware that this is not a linear process, rather, it is akin to walking a labyrinth. As we head toward the centre, we can feel as if we are moving away from it. It's easy to feel despondent and default back to the old circuitry. The key to entrenching the new pathway is to keep catching the old behaviour and gently guide ourselves back. Once again, courage, support and realignment with value systems and compassion for yourself are required here.

6. *Practice*: The process of change requires perseverance, practice and commitment to self. More than all that, it requires patience and support. Practically speaking, I find that making time to plan helps us to create a loose structure and support to make the changes easier. For example, this could mean redesigning your physical environment, planning your meals so you have the necessary ingredients. Planning actually saves time and energy and supports us to make the changes we are making. When we feel overwhelmed and tired, we tend to default to old patterns, so we need to have our strategies in place when this

happens. I also find the idea of 'habit stacking', described by SJ Scott in his book *Habit Stacking*, quite useful and interesting. Basically, this is about stitching the new habit onto a habit that is already there. In other words, you are piggy-backing off a neural pathway you have already created to save yourself from creating a new one. For example, you would like to take a vitamin supplement but you always forget. You could use something that is already a habit as a reminder to take it, for example, after brushing your teeth.

'Nerves that fire together wire together', so the more the skill, habits, behaviour, feelings and emotions are practised, the more deeply the neural pathways will be entrenched. In response, new receptors become switched on and primed on the surface of the cells and the physical body begins to transform. In my 15 years' experience of working with the mind–body connection I have hundreds of examples of people who have healed their physical ailments and completely changed their relationship to life and themselves by working through this process.

7. *The shift*: This is when new neural pathways have become deeply embedded and the new habit is permanent. The entire body–mind system has become rewired to create a new habit or way of living and being. This is the 'new normal'. The software of the subconscious mind has been reprogrammed. While the old programme will probably rear its head every now and again, it passes quickly as the new default programme sets in. This, however, requires constant awareness and vigilance. By now, the skill of mindfulness has become more finely tuned.

Consider the habits of thoughts, feelings and behaviour that might be depleting your energy system. Is there one small thing that you could work on reprogramming? Go through the 7 steps. Where do you think you are?

Studies are showing that it actually takes about 55 days of daily practice to create a new habit. Experts in the field of sports science suggests we need 2000 repeated actions to embed the pathway. We may not know for sure, the process is layered, but what we do know for sure is that change is possible. We just have to remember why we're doing it in the first place.

Our ability to grow, adapt and change is what makes being human truly amazing and wonderful.

> Energy Formula
> *Commitment + practice + patience + support*
> *= new neural pathways = authentic energy*

CHAPTER 13

How belief systems affect energy

Belief systems are the way we relate to the world; the lens through which we perceive our reality.

THAMI'S STORY: BREAD AND BELIEFS
Name: Thami Selebi
Age: 39
Character traits: Open mindedness, difficulty receiving support
Life-changing experiences: Grandmother's death
Stress catalysts in last two years: Moving from his home town to Johannesburg
Stress Indicators: Binge drinking, gambling, heartburn, heart palpitations
Presentation on energy zone map: Burnout zone

He closed his eyes and took a long deep breath. Bread. Bread in the oven. Suddenly he was a child again, sitting at the yellow, mottled panelyte table in his grandmother's kitchen, his mouth watering at the thought of taking his first bite into the crusty end that Gogo cut especially for him, thick melting butter seeping over the edges. The memory was that of a soft blanket that brought comfort in the scary dark place in which he had found himself. 'This place can't be so bad if they're baking homemade bread,' Thami thought to himself.

Thami had been dealing with heart palpitations for the last few months and night sweats that had left his sheets drenched even in the dry chilly nights of the Johannesburg winter. One night it all came to a head, the searing pain across his chest left him breathless. He was convinced he was having a heart attack. He anticipated seeing the proverbial white light at the end of the tunnel as the ambulance weaved through the sparse traffic to the emergency room, but the ECG and the blood tests were clear. There was no myocardial infarction, just a panic attack. The psychiatrist on call diagnosed Thami with anxiety disorder and depression. Depression? He was perplexed. He would have preferred it to be a heart attack.

Despite vehement protests and violent threats, Thami agreed to book into the mental wellness facility that specialised in depression and anxiety, for four weeks. He felt like the ultimate failure. He had succumbed to weakness. After three weeks of individual counselling, group therapy and a cocktail of antidepressants, anxiolytics, mood stabilisers and sleeping pills, Thami decided that he had had enough. Enough of people convincing him that he was depressed and enough of the drugs that made him feel like a walking zombie. He was stressed. He was overworking. His boss was unreasonable. It was simple. His girlfriend had threatened that if he discharged himself, she would leave him. He had had enough of her too.

Bonini, his girlfriend, had heard from a friend that there was a doctor who was treating people with natural alternatives and minimal medication. She took the liberty of making the appointment for Thami to see me.

It was a sunny but crisp day in June. I met a tall, good-looking man with eyes that spoke of some inner turmoil. He seemed desperate and despairing at the same time. He was accompanied by Bonini, a friendly, small-framed woman with a confident handshake. Thami relayed his story in a bored, matter-of-fact way. He said that after 21 days of being on his medication, he didn't feel any better and had decided not to fill his repeat prescription. He was curious to see how he felt without it. It seemed to me that his anxiety was hiding between the layers of agitation and frustration, and the room felt heavy with the words he was not saying. He appeared lost and confused, struggling to accept this diagnosis of depression. Black men don't get depressed. It's a 'white man's sickness'. That's what he said. That's what he thought.

At the time, Thami was living in a small town called Mahikeng in the North West province of South Africa, where he had spent his childhood years. He felt drawn to moving back after his divorce, four years previously. He was seeking the simplicity of home. He grew up in a Christian home with the strong values of honesty, humility and simplicity as life's guiding principles. Johannesburg had robbed him of that. And a lot more.

His life in Johannesburg was fast and furious. He and his then wife had been living the high life; shoes and shopping, canapés and convertibles. It just felt wrong. Wealth in his eyes equated with arrogance and materialism. Value systems had somehow got tangled and they got divorced. Thami shared his experience of his messy and complicated marriage, how he agonised over the feeling that he was not living in integrity with his values. This is what really kept him up at night. He kept his thoughts and feelings deeply buried for a long time until he could no longer access them, let alone share them with someone else. Work was the perfect distraction while partying it up with his friends and gambling filled the gap over the weekends. The deeper he buried his head in the sand, the more suffocated and disconnected he felt. The more disconnected he felt, the more he distracted himself. And so the cycle continued.

Initially, the distraction of work did wonders for his career. He was thriving on adrenalised energy. He exceeded the company's expectations of him and was promoted to marketing manager of the bread-making company. Working there had ignited a childhood passion for bread and opened his eyes to a niche in his community back home. He used his time at the company to study and hone the craft of bread making. But slowly, the anxiety began to spill over and the sleepless nights took their toll. Heated clashes with his wife became almost a daily occurrence to the point where he had no energy left to muster up a logical argument. He went silent instead. His anger gave way to despair and his dream got lost in confusion and divorce papers.

After the divorce went through, Thami craved the comfort of his home town, but his move back to Mahikeng was disappointing. He accepted a job as marketing manager of a nondescript local radio station, but instead of freeing him, it suffocated him – the docile lifestyle, the complacency, the boxed thinking and stale way of living. Nothing had changed in 15 years. Everything felt stuck. He felt stuck. And exhausted.

Thami's narrative was layered with strong ideas and steadfast opinions about how the world worked, what was important, and what wasn't, what was right and what was wrong. His worldview was structured and binary, ebony and ivory. To him the world was a fickle and unsafe place where he always had to watch his back, because someone was sure to put a knife in it. He believed that whatever he was going through, he needed to sort himself out, because he was a strong, tough and capable man. I found Thami to be bright and insightful and he easily followed my train of thought as we examined how his belief systems, both conscious and unconscious, were feeding his narrative, his neurobiological response to them and, ultimately, his health. If he was serious about taking charge of his life, he had no choice but to dig deep and do the hard work of examining the belief systems that were no longer working to support his best life.

Belief systems are the way we relate to the world; the lens through which we perceive our reality. They are fundamental to shaping our value systems and informing our choices. Many of the beliefs we hold are clear. We know what they are and we endeavour to live by them. They are our anchors for our journey through life. Other belief systems may not be so clear or conscious, or may no longer be valid. They lurk in the shadows of our psyche and feed thought and behaviour patterns that constantly trigger the stress response. They feed our voice of judgement, fear and criticism.

We extracted some core beliefs from Thami's story that were feeding his thoughts, feelings and behaviour. The belief that 'Black people don't get depressed' was a belief formed by the stereotype that 'depression' was a condition of the privileged, and that it belonged to the world of excess and materialism. It was a first world problem, a 'white woman's disease'. In the world that he came from, there were more fundamental issues that needed to be addressed. This fed into another core belief, that of 'I am strong and therefore I don't need support'. These beliefs prevented Thami from recognising that what he was experiencing was real, and prevented him from seeking support when he needed it. It had fed behaviour that had ultimately caused him to end up in an emergency room. Even when he did end up at the mental wellness treatment facility, the belief that 'I can't trust anyone' made him choose to play his cards close to his chest. He was very cautious about sharing personal information with people he hardly knew. His discomfort around his big city lifestyle was driven by a values and beliefs system that became enmeshed and confused. His value system of honesty, integrity, passion and desire for simplicity somehow became blurred by his belief that 'money equates arrogance' and 'rich people are superficial'. Did these beliefs cause him to miss opportunities that could have been a stepping stone to following his true passion of setting up community-based bakeries? Did his voice of judgement cause him to create his own obstacles? Would he have made different choices if he had adapted his beliefs and changed his perspective on certain issues?

Belief systems become problematic when they become fixed and rigid. They narrow our perspective and become a way in which we set ourselves up for disappointment and frustration. The more fixed and rigid our belief systems, the more expectation we build up around the way we think the world should work. Imagine the chemical cocktail of stress hormones that brews in our system on a daily basis when the world does not fit into our worldview? At the time, he had no idea at a conscious level of what was happening inside him. His belief systems were still underneath the radar.

All he was aware of was that he was unhappy and frustrated. Belief systems are especially dangerous when they lurk under the surface of our conscious awareness and when they seem contrary to logic. For example, Thami's belief that 'I don't trust anyone' was not conscious, yet showed up very clearly in his behaviour. Somewhere along the line in his life, he had the experience of trust being betrayed. It could have been the smallest thing that evoked a strong emotional response or a major life event that shook up his entire family dynamic. Whatever the case, an association was made between trust and betrayal, and a neural pathway laid down fact-linked fear, lack of trust, emotional suppression and defensiveness. This, in turn, fed anxiety and his behaviour of overworking and drinking with friends or zoning out in front of the television. Subconscious belief systems also display parasite behaviour. They lurk in the shadows, feed off our energy and attract the situations and experiences that reinforce them. This way they keep themselves fed and alive. A good example of this is a time when Thami let his guard down, and in a vulnerable moment shared his feelings with his wife, which she used as 'ammunition' in another argument. That reinforced his belief that 'no one can be trusted'.

It wasn't easy for Thami to recognise some of his belief systems but in facing some hard truths in the session, he began to drop his defensiveness and his jaw began to soften. Through sharing his story with me, he was already challenging some very deeply held beliefs around trust and support, and was amazed at how relieved and energised he was already feeling.

A week later, Thami returned. He had given a great deal of thought to his life and some of the belief systems that governed his thinking and choices. He discovered that he had some very positive belief systems such as 'you can achieve anything you set your mind to' but also needed to watch out for that dreaded line 'I'm not good enough' and 'fear of failure'. This is almost a collective belief. That week, while still on leave, I encouraged Thami to journal his thoughts. The process of writing reignited his creativity, reminded him of his passion. He closed his eyes and took a deep breath. Bread.

I never saw Thami for another session. I'm not sure how his journey unfolded or if he ever set up his community-based bakeries back in his home town. He did refer many people to me though, so I believe something must have happened for him in those sessions.

Understanding belief systems

Belief systems work is a core aspect of my integrated approach to health and energy management. It strikes at the core of what drives our thought patterns, feelings and habits. If we are truly committed to creating positive change in our lives, at some point we will be faced with examining and working with our beliefs and questioning what has shaped them. In the last few years, there have been some fascinating studies done in the field of belief systems and how they relate to our bodies. Bruce Lipton outlines his research and sheds light on his amazing findings in his groundbreaking book *The Biology of Belief*. He writes that most of our belief systems are actually formed in the first seven years of life. In these formative years, our brain waves correspond to being in a hypnotic trance. We are in this trance for most of our childhood, downloading information, storing it and creating massive amounts of neural pathways around it. We create beliefs around much of what we see and experience, especially if that experience has a strong emotional charge. We also form beliefs based on what we have been taught around good and bad, right and wrong, the kind of behaviour that is acceptable and the kind that goes against societal norms. We are conditioned through the collective beliefs of society and through those held by our parents. Recent research has shown that we can even inherit belief systems on a cellular level through our ancestors!

Sometimes the work of unravelling our beliefs is a complex and layered process and requires constant self-reflection. But it can also happen in a second, where the recognition in itself is a letting go. Not all of our belief systems need to be shed, though. Some are valuable and support our growth, and are in integrity with who we are. We need to be aware of these too and focus on building the neural pathways around these. These belief systems are the good kind, and support a feeling of empowerment, meaning and authentic energy.

How do we go about the work of figuring out what our belief systems are, especially if they are unconscious? It begins with mindfulness; the present-moment awareness of what we react to and how we react to it. Eventually we will begin to see patterns of behaviour emerging. We tend to react in the same way to the same things in a habitual way. We will also soon start to see that we have the same kind of thoughts around the situation, because we perceive it in a certain way. We see the world through the lens of our belief. Take Thami's case. He saw the world through his lens of 'I'm not good enough'. He would make assumptions about others' behaviour, and would take everything personally, even though, in reality, his perception of the situation was no further from the truth. For example, when his boss was irritable, or when someone was yawning in a presentation, Thami's reality was that he was messing up.

To begin the process of freeing yourself from limiting beliefs, make yourself a cup of tea, grab a journal and take yourself through this process of recognising, identifying and finally let go..

Mindfulness of belief – four steps

1. *Identifying your core beliefs*: Begin by identifying where you are on the energy zone map. Make a list of your current symptoms from the map. Name some of your habits and behaviours that could be causing these symptoms, such as taking on too much, difficulty saying no, addictions, skipping meals, not resting enough, overworking. Name your everyday range of feelings, for example, frustration, guilt, irritation, disappointment, feeling burdened, feeling overwhelmed.

    Make a list of the most common triggers for these feelings – what or who activates these feelings?

What kind of thoughts do you have about these situations? How do you perceive them? What is the story that you build up around these situations? Do they centre on judgements, assumptions, resentment, taking things personally?

This process will help you to uncover some of the beliefs that could drive your feelings and behaviour. These are some common belief systems that we carry:
- I'm different and never fit it.
- Every time I open my heart to someone I get hurt.
- I am alone in the world.
- No matter what I do it is never good enough.
- I'm not good enough.
- If I haven't found my life purpose, I have failed.
- I can only be happy if I have a partner.
- If people really knew me, they wouldn't love me.
- You have to fight to get ahead in this world.
- Everything will fall apart if I don't take charge.
- This bubble of happiness, joy or success is going to burst.
- My husband/wife/partner betrayed me.
- I'm always right.
- No one ever considers my needs.
- People only look out for themselves.
- I'll be happy when I'm rich.
- Money is not important.
- Spiritual people shouldn't be rich.
- People can't be trusted.
- If I don't do it no one will.

2. *Where does this belief come from?*: Reflect on how this belief could have been formed. Can you remember what shaped this belief? Was it created through something you experienced or witnessed? Is it something you were taught or conditioned to believe? Is this belief yours or have you inherited it? Often we are not sure what has created a particular belief.

3. *Does it work for me?*: Reflect on whether this belief system actually works for you. Does it support your life or does it create stress and anxiety? Which beliefs would you like to let

go of or reshape? Sometimes a certain belief that has supported us in the past and given us the drive to move past obstacles and struggle has become irrelevant and is causing more harm than good.
4. *Letting it go*: Each time we see, hear or experience something that pulls us away from a state of calm and balance, or the second we react to something, we need to develop the ability to stop and examine our emotional reaction to the situation, our thoughts about it, and the core belief systems that underpin them.

   Practise the ABC formula:
   - **Awareness**: Become mindful of when you have been triggered and how it feels in your body. What sensations do you feel in your body when something has shifted you from a state of balance?
   - Breathing into it: Use your breath to slow down to move out of reactive mode and ask yourself:
     - What thought did I have related to that situation?
     - How have I interpreted the situation?
     - What belief system has been activated?
   - Conscious choice:
     - Can I choose to see the situation differently and let it go?
     - Does this situation require me to consciously communicate something?
     - Can I channel this adrenalised energy into something else?

   The activation of belief systems and the neural pathways connected to our thoughts, feelings and behaviours are probably the biggest activator of our adrenalised energy and reactive response. It is for this reason that I have included it here. Let's not assume that by reading this chapter you're going to uncover and unravel all your negative beliefs in a short space of time. Remember, this is a lifetime's work and takes patience and commitment to yourself. We can't always make sense of them ourselves, but at least we can begin to open our awareness to some of the deeper factors that lie at the root of energy depletion and burnout, and we can commit to a process of deeper self-enquiry. It's a fascinating, liberating and energising journey!

> Energy Formula
> *Awareness of (behaviour + feeling + thought)/belief system + conscious choice = authentic energy*

Heart Intelligence

CHAPTER 14

Emotions and energy

We develop all kinds of unconscious mechanisms and strategies to hold onto the good and avoid the bad that we eventually disconnect from the healthy expression of emotion all together.

CARLO'S STORY: ENERGY IN MOTION
Name: Carlo Greco
Age: 71
Character traits: Generosity, stubbornness
Life changing experiences: Mother's death and moving to South Africa
Stress catalysts in last two years: Stroke
Stress indicators: Being non-compliant in taking medication, depression
Presentation on energy zone map: Burnout zone

Carlo felt most calm at dusk, when the last of the sunrays made the trees glow and the evening's meal in the oven merged with the scent of jasmine from the garden. From the time that he first arrived in South Africa, a decade after the war, taking an early evening stroll had become a ritual. All those years ago when he was filled with hope and life held promise, breathing in the fresh African air was energising. These days, even though the stroke left him with a subtle limp, his walk among the trees in the transient moments of twilight still offered Carlo a sense of stillness and peace.

Carlo was born in a small village in northern Italy. His father was a builder and stalwart member of the community. He had lost his older brother in the war which had left his mother emotionally volatile and completely unpredictable. In moments of vulnerability he allowed himself to soften and receive her nurturing and motherly love. But most of the time he would be hiding in the shadows, holding his breath in anticipation of the next outburst of venomous anger that left the house feeling dark for days. Work opportunities in the neighbouring towns became the perfect excuse for his father to escape, so Carlo bore the brunt of his mother's erratic moods. He spoke little and became hypervigilant for the signs that his mother was about to have an emotional outburst. He developed a way to cope by retreating into his inner world of thought, dreams and imagination.

He was just 12 years old when his mother died of cancer. He remembers standing at her grave among the villagers all donned in black, feeling nothing. A few years after his mother's death, Carlo's father decided to follow the wave of immigrants that were settling in South Africa. At that time, South African industries were booming, and there was a great demand for the kind of skill his father had. At the age of 17, he arrived in a strange foreign land at the southern tip of Africa, not speaking a word of English. Within three years, he was speaking English fluently, had a steady job and was engaged to a beautiful girl from a big Italian family. They made a great team; Lorenza was outspoken, practical and hardworking; Carlo was ambitious and focused. A house and two children later, their little family was complete. Life had begun.

Carlo was a man of foresight, fiercely independent and focused. Before long, he quit his job and started his own business. It grew exponentially. He sold his house and built a bigger one on a small holding just outside Johannesburg. To anyone watching from the outside, it would have seemed that Carlo had it all. A loving family, a successful business and a home that was always abundant with family and food. He travelled, read books and enjoyed meaningful conversations. Many were drawn to his warmth and generosity. So he just gave more. Through the years, as his hair silvered and his face wrinkled he became even more magnetic, a Robert de Niro look alike, some would say. But for Carlo this was never enough.

He spent his life creating contingency plans for a thousand worst-case scenarios that never happened. The more he created and built, the more he feared losing it. Fear took on the form of anxiety, anxiety took on the form of physical tension. Eventually, fear had buried itself so deeply in his body that he didn't even know it was there. When his sons decided to go to university and not to join his business, Carlo was angry, disappointed and heavy with futility. What legacy would he leave behind? What had he spent his whole life building if this was to be the outcome? But all these questions stayed locked in his heart – never properly felt, never expressed. He dealt with it like he had dealt with everything else. He created another plan, formulated another strategy. He would find a buyer for his business, sell the small holding, scale down his life, and enjoy an eternal summer by spending half the year in Italy.

One day, Carlo was sitting in his favourite armchair after his walk. Marco, his grandson, had brought him a cup of tea and he was settling in to watch his favourite programme on the National Geographic channel. In a flash, his world went black and frozen. Marco called out to his grandad but there was no response. Carlo had suffered a stroke. The scan showed a coin-sized grey shadow on the left side of his brain. Fortunately, it wasn't the kind of stroke caused by a haemorrhage, which is the worst kind. He got medical attention soon enough and the damage to his brain tissue was minimised.

In the weeks that followed, Carlo felt raw, vulnerable and exposed. His words fell out, tumbled and slurred, and his leg felt like a heavy log disconnected from the rest of his body. For Lorenza and the children, the most startling change was that for the very first time, they witnessed their father shedding tears. Carlo wept tears of gratitude for the love that surrounded him, felt deep regret for all the words unspoken, grief for a part of himself that he feared he had lost forever.

I saw Carlo every fortnight for a check in and blood tests to monitor his blood levels. It was remarkable to watch his recovery process. Through a rehab regime of physiotherapy, breath work and massages, Carlo regained his strength. His limp and speech improved and he returned to the office. It was business as usual. But the foundation of Carlo's world had fundamentally shifted. He had to learn to navigate through a new unfamiliar landscape of unfiltered feelings and emotion. Feelings for which he didn't have the vocabulary.

On some days, his eyes sparkled with humour and mischief, and on other days they told a different story. Although Carlo still wasn't able to find words for what he was feeling, what had fundamentally shifted in him was his capacity to feel and express his emotions. His inner world felt richer as his relationships deepened, softened and became more real. It was as if the stroke had shattered the armour that Carlo had unconsciously created as a protective mechanism from a very early age. This internalisation of his emotions became his strategy to keep his world safe and controlled, but eventually this caused a pattern of suppression that created a chronic build-up of tension and inflammation in his system. Ironically, the stroke gave him back the gift of vulnerability, his ability to feel and, in a strange way, a big part of his humanity.

The complexities of human emotion

I have always been intrigued by the complexities of human emotion, its role in our lives and impact on our health. In fact, it was my observation of the obvious link between emotion and physical symptoms in my early years as a GP that fuelled my deeper enquiry into body–mind medicine. I saw patients' deep rage show up as depression or fibromyalgia, I saw how anxiety was linked to irritable bowel syndrome and insomnia, and how deep-seated fear underpinned so many illnesses. Over the years I began to see the patterns emerging in my patients between their physical symptoms and what was going on in their lives. The more time I took to listen to their stories, the more obvious this connection became. I felt compelled to deepen my enquiry into this body–mind phenomenon and think about a new way of practising my craft.

My curiosity led me to some cutting-edge information, including the intriguing work of neuroscientist Dr Candice Pert, who through her research has shown how emotions are chemical information systems that link our body and mind. Her research confirms what I have always suspected: chronic suppression of our emotions creates a massive disruption to the balance of our physiology and can have potentially devastating effects on our immune system and ability to dampen inflammatory processes in the tissues. This can eventually lead to a whole host of medical conditions including cancer, autoimmune disorders and chronic fatigue. The conundrum, however, is that in as much as feeling and expression of emotion is important and necessary for optimum health and energy, our nature as humans is to avoid pain or 'negative' feelings at all cost and to hold onto the 'positive or happy feelings' for dear life. We develop all kinds of unconscious mechanisms and strategies to hold onto the good and avoid the bad that we eventually disconnect from the healthy expression of emotion all together.

On the most primal level, emotions are energy states that have been programmed into our system as a mechanism for survival, but they are also there to deepen our connection to each other, foster empathy, fuel creativity, instigate inner enquiry, bring meaning and deepen our capacity for joy.

Fear protects us from danger and activates the survival-based fight–flight response to which we have frequently referred. Anger helps us to create boundaries and fight injustice. Sadness deepens empathy and connection with each other. Joy makes us feel alive. Emotions are dynamic states of energy and catalysts to action, movement and change. Even the word 'e-motion' explains itself – 'energy in motion'. Each of the six basic emotions of anger, fear, sadness, happiness, surprise and disgust are linked to the release of different peptides or chemicals that effect the very specific changes in our cells, which each have a specific representation in the amygdala. In other words, each of the core emotional states can be differentiated by its psychophysiological reactions and autonomic functions. One of the most profound examples of this is the research done on tears, which reveals that the chemical composition of happy tears differs to that of sad tears!

When an emotion has been activated by an internal or external trigger, we experience a heightened energy state, which is an opening or doorway to an action or awareness. If we consciously or unconsciously suppress this energy and stand in the way of its natural expression, it gets locked into our tissues, sending stress signals back to the brain and pushing us into the danger zone. Either that or it builds up like a pressure cooker until we explode through an amygdala hijack.

The modern view of emotions is that they occur in two phases. An emotion will be activated through the sensory processing and interpretation of an external event in comparison against pre-existing memories stored in the hippocampus, the brain's memory bank. When the interpretation of a current event matches the emotional memory of a past event, it will trigger the same emotion as the original event. This initial 'fast track response' and the biochemical and physical chemical changes that occur at lightning speed lasts for around two minutes. If we can allow the full expression of the emotion, the emotion will subside and we will return to baseline. However, usually the full expression of the feeling is not appropriate or comfortable and the brain gets involved to moderate the feeling. This happens in conjunction with the 'slow track' of emotion, which is fed by the thoughts that we have related to the emotion as well as the feedback that the brain receives from the heart, muscles, neurotransmitters in the bowel, muscles and breathing pattern in response to the initial emotion.

For example, Lorenza is upset that Carlo has forgotten to book the plane tickets for their next trip to Italy and raises her voice in frustration. Lorenza's words and pitch of her voice are interpreted and compared against an unconscious past memory of Carlo's mother shouting and insulting him. Carlo feels the flush in his face and his body tensing up as his adrenal glands release stress hormones. If Carlo allowed the natural full expression of this feeling in this moment, he would scream, or beat a pillow, or do something to vent or release his anger. But Carlo instead keeps himself in check and internalises the anger. His thoughts about the situation further feed into the slow track as his muscles tense up, breathing pattern becomes shallow and heart rate quickens. The slow track can last for a long time, either until the energy of the emotion builds up to a point of explosion, or gets deeply internalised creating a chronic activation of the stress response. Now we can see how over time this can lead to disease.

Consciously tending to our emotional landscape is the greatest key to managing our energy state. But often it is not easy to name the primary emotion that is at the root of the feelings that we experience in a typical day, which are usually versions of the core emotion or mixed emotions. For example, frustration is fear in a form of anger that has no outlet, while irritation is a mild version of anger. Guilt is a mixture of sadness and fear, and anxiety is another form of fear, as is worry. While the mind is interpreting our feelings state as irritation or frustration, the neurochemistry is the same. The body activates the same biochemical response to irritation as it would to anger. In other words, the brain can't differentiate between the core emotion and its watered-down version, and so its effect on the body will be the same.

We are also really good at masking one feeling with another that is easier to feel. Or we use one emotion as a way to cope with another. It is easier to feel anger than sadness. I often come across people who seem angry on the surface but underneath hold a deeply buried sadness that they can't access. I believe that each of us has a default feeling of emotion that becomes our emotional set point or neural pathway, a core emotion that in early life was triggered most intensely. The neural pathway becomes deeply entrenched for that particular feeling. For example, a child who lost a parent at an early age could have felt deep sadness and as a result the neural pathway for sadness became most deeply entrenched. Later in life, that child grows to have an increased sensitivity to experiences that trigger sadness and in the process entrenches the pathway even further. In Carlo's case, his default core emotion could be fear experienced as anxiety. This doesn't mean that we don't all feel the full range of emotions, just that we are more prone to feeling a particular emotion and that we can filter all our emotions into that neural pathway.

There has also been a great amount of debate in neuroscience circles around what comes first, a thought or emotion. Do thoughts feed emotions or do emotions trigger thoughts? Recent discoveries on the bioenergy field around the heart has also thrown a spanner in the works for this debate. Research is indicating that the bioelectrical activity generated by the heart rhythm sends the signals to the emotional centre in the brain. This implies that our physical heart might in fact be the source of our feelings.

The bottom line, however, is that the body, mind and heart all operate as one biodynamic interconnected information system and, in order to use the energy of our emotions efficiently and effectively, we need to get comfortable with them, be able to name them and get to understand what they are showing us, and most importantly, learn to express them in a healthy way. We have been so conditioned to keeping our feelings in check that they become distorted and toxic in the process. We have found a way for emotion to bypass our awareness by going straight into the head which is really good at dissection, analysis, processing and finding solutions, which in turn adds more fuel to the fire. In the process we bypass the vital step of feeling and expressing.

Healthy expression of feelings is one of the most energising and liberating experiences. Having a good cry can be so deeply therapeutic and a crucial way to release healing, yet we avoid it at all costs. We feel embarrassed and ashamed by our tears or apologise as tears well up. Brene Brown, a research professor and storyteller, in her bestselling book *Rising Strong* and in her popular TedX talk 'The Power of Vulnerability', shares her compelling research on this subject. She speaks about tending to our emotional life in terms of vulnerability and the courage that it requires to live a life that is richer, healthier and more meaningful. The popularity of her work reveals our collective need for permission and validation of what makes us most human. We have become so good at bypassing the heart and over-intellectualising our feelings that all our channels of emotional expression become rusty from disuse, to the point that we even suppress joy. I have witnessed how destructive suppressed joy can become.

I love the work of Madan Kataria, an Indian physician who popularised laughter as a form of exercise. Some studies have demonstrated that laughter may increase pain threshold and increase endorphin release which promotes social bonding.

One of the greatest gifts that my mother gave me was permission to express my feelings without being ashamed of them. I have a particular memory of when I was a little girl of five or six and I was crying. Wailing in fact. Instead of pacifying me with a typical 'don't cry', she opened up a chocolate instead, with a soft mint centre, made a little cup with the foil wrapper, held it under my eyes and told me to 'collect my tears'. It was such a poignant moment and one I will never forget.

How do we begin to go about using emotions as the energising force they are meant to be? The reality is that while emotions are raw and primal we have the ability, through attention and conscious awareness, to use our emotions constructively for the purpose of growth, energy and meaning. As Candace Pert so eloquently puts it in her book, *Molecules of Emotions*, 'All emotions are healthy. Anger, fear, sadness, the so-called negative emotions, are as healthy as peace, courage and joy. All honest emotions are positive emotions.'

Mastering energy in motion

1. **Reflection exercise:** Take a few moments to reflect on the following two questions:
   - What is your default mechanism or strategy that you have developed to deal with your emotions?
     - Suppression with food, alcohol, smoking, medication, drugs
     - Avoidance and distraction of work, keeping busy, music
     - Over intellectualisation or 'analysis paralysis'
     - Projection onto others or a system of blame or criticism
     - Spiritual bypass, i.e., use of spiritual methods or concepts to avoid feeling
     - Self-destruction, e.g., self-mutilation, cutting, pulling out hair
   - How are your emotions eventually expressed?
     - Physical symptoms or illness
     - Emotional outbursts (amygdala hijacks)
     - Obsessive compulsive behaviour
     - Navigating your emotional landscape
2. **Apply the ABC formula**
   - **Awareness**
     - Catch the drift.
     - Notice that you have been activated or triggered or have drifted away from your Stillpoint or sense of peace.
     - Name the emotion.
     - Try to get a sense of the core emotion. You might not always be able to identify it.
     - Identify through the body. The sensations we feel in our body give us a clue. For example:
       Sadness: lump in throat, tightness in chest, general tiredness and low energy
       Anger: muscle tension especially around the head and neck area, clenched jaws, build-up of heat in face; increase in heart rate; holding the breath. The body is preparing to fight.

Fear/Excitement: feeling of 'butterflies in the stomach', as the fight–flight response kicks in and blood is quickly shunted away from the digestive system; increased heart rate and respiratory rate, dry mouth, sweating

Happiness/Joy: an effervescent energy all over the body

- Identify through your thoughts. Sometimes the thought that you are having about a situation will help you to identify the emotion.

- **Breathing**
  - Once you have named the emotion or feeling, let yourself feel it, not feed it. In other words, deepen your experience of the feeling by using the breath to open up into it. This is where the courage to be vulnerable comes in.
  - Use your breath to move out of the reactive, suppressive, avoidance or analysis mode, which may be your normal reaction. Instead of shutting down, open up. Do this by breathing into the actual physical sensation and exhale with a soft sigh or a prolonged exhalation.

- **Conscious choice**

  After we have connected with the emotion and experienced it, we are ready to bring the mind to make a conscious choice about what to do with the energy of the emotion.
  - *Communicate it*: Perhaps your anger is justified and appropriate and is guiding you to take action towards a situation that needs to be changed. This could mean that you need to communicate something to someone. However, when you have slowed down your reaction and owned the feeling, you are more ready to communicate it in a clear and more responsive way. For example, you will achieve a far better outcome from giving yourself space to breathe before reacting to an email that has really triggered your anger.
  - *Change your thought or perception*: Very often, the emotion that we feel is triggered by an interpretation of a situation or an assumption you have made, which may not be true at all. Changing the thought or allowing yourself

to see the situation from another angle will change how you feel about it. However, this will only work once you have allowed yourself to feel the original feeling. It is a common strategy to slap a 'positive thought' onto an unexpressed feeling, which is like stitching an infected wound.
- Release it.
- Cry or laugh.
- Write or paint.
- Talk to a friend who won't over analyse, judge or feed your story.
- Exercise.
    The energy of emotion is stored on a somatic level. Moving the body and breathing is an effective way to release stuck emotion.
- Harness and direct it.
    Through this process, the emotion might have revealed or opened your mind to something that needs to change, or an action that needs to be taken. Grab hold of it, gather it up and direct it in the direction of constructive action. Use the emotion as fuel for action.
- Be with it.
    Sometimes we have no idea why we feel a certain way and none of the above methods work to come back to a state of equilibrium. In this case, just let yourself be with it, honouring its presence and knowing that it will pass. Once again, remember to feel it, not feed it. The insight will reveal itself at a later stage.

3. **Tending to your emotional landscape**
In order to skillfully navigate through our emotional landscape and enjoy it, we need to tend to it as we would with any garden.
Diet: Eating a wholesome nourishing diet will provide your body with enough vitamins, minerals, essential fatty acids and amino acids to produce healthy levels of neurotransmitters that will help stabilise your moods. The latest research has shown the link between good gut flora and healthy emotions.

Exercise: The mind resides in the whole body. Exercise not only helps us to release the stuck emotion from the tissue but also helps the production of mood-stabilising hormones. We need to exercise in a way that balances both energising cortisol and calming serotonin.

Mindfulness: Dedicate 10–12 minutes of a mindfulness practice daily, which develops the ability to simply watch thoughts and feelings without reacting to it. It will also help you to identify belief systems, thought patterns and habits that keep emotion stuck.

Breathing: The HeartMath foundation has done extensive research on the role of conscious breathing to change the heart rate variability and heart coherence, which in turn charges the electromagnetic field around the heart. We now know that there are more nerve fibres from the heart to the brain than the brain to the heart, which in effect means that the brain listens to the heart! Refer to David O' Hare's 365 technique mentioned in chapter 5. Breathe in for five seconds and out for five seconds, three times a day, for five minutes at a time.

Receive: Replenish your heart energy through being nurtured, connecting with others who inspire and support you, spend time in nature. Allocate enough time to anything that inspires you: music, art, books, movies and people.

> Energy Formula
> *Naming + (feeling - feeding) + expressing = authentic energy*

CHAPTER 15

Applying boundaries

Constantly saying 'yes' becomes a habit and pattern, even an addiction. A benchmark is created and we teach others how to treat us.

> **MARILYN'S STORY: BOUNDARY TO BOUNDFREE**
> **Name:** Marilyn Parkinson
> **Age:** 48
> **Character traits:** Integrity, self-doubt
> **Life-changing experiences:** Leaving home to work abroad
> **Stress catalysts in last two years:** Building her business
> **Stress indicators:** Irritability, weight gain
> **Presentation on energy zone map:** Burnout zone

It was her little secret. She had been debating it for months. She hadn't breathed a word of it to anyone in case they dissuaded her and ridiculed her idea as part of a middle-aged existential crisis. But for Marilyn, the tattoo was a symbol of liberation and of reclaiming a part of her identity that had become buried under the burden of adulthood and responsibility. She held out her arm and looked away as the pen oozed ink into her skin. The feeling was not what she had anticipated. It was like the sensation of deep scratches more than the sharp pain of skin being pierced. For the first time since she was 23, Marilyn felt exhilarated.

Marilyn grew up with Table Mountain as her backdrop and the Beatles and Rolling Stones as the soundtrack to her life. In those years, South Africa was volatile, uncertain and suffocating, cut off and sanctioned by most of the Western world. Marilyn was enraged by the apartheid system which she felt a part of and just wanted to escape it all. After university, when her brother was sent to the army, Marilyn believed that exploring the world would open her mind to the greater possibilities for her life. London was the logical safe place to start. Her aunt lived there so if she was stranded she would have a place to go. Like many, Marilyn found London energising and depressing, depending on the season. Winters were harsh and dampened her spirit. The waitressing job was hard work and paid little, but at least it would pay for her next stop, which she hoped would be Paris, the city of her dreams. But months after living and working in London, Marilyn fell in love. And as luck would have it, with a South African. Long before she had anticipated, she found herself back in South Africa, planning her wedding.

When the children were born, she made a conscious decision to put her career aspirations on hold while focusing on raising her young children. She didn't ever want to feel torn between work and home, or guilty for not giving her family enough attention. But when her daughters were well settled in their primary school routine, she believed that the time had come to focus on doing something that stirred her passion while contributing to the rising household expenses.

Over the years, she played around with a few business ideas from importing clothing from India to running a funky coffee shop. She even started a bespoke children's clothing range, which serendipitously led her to an idea that really excited her and that leveraged her business background and flair for creativity.

People loved the idea of a children's party events company with a difference, one that catered delicious and healthy treats and that provided entertainment too. It was a slow start, but with hard work and persistence it grew steadily. Coming up with new creative ideas was energising and rewarding. The business provided the perfect balance between meaningful work and quality time with her family. But as her business grew so did her expenses. Between managing bookings and enquiries, organising the logistics for the parties and managing her accounts, she found herself working later and later into the night. She wasn't willing to compromise afternoon time with her children. She was clear about her choice to have that time exclusively dedicated to them, even if it meant that work was put on hold for that time.

The reality, however, was that she still felt a deep sense of responsibility to her business and clients. It just wasn't in her to do a job that was less than perfect. If her plans for an event in any way veered from her original vision, which included every last detail down to the way the serviettes were placed, it caused a great deal of anxiety and sleepless nights. But Marilyn forged on, working later into the nights and functioning on less sleep. Extracting herself from bed was more of an effort, so the morning routine became more rushed and frenetic. She noticed herself becoming more ratty and irritable with her children, which in turn triggered a whole cycle of guilt. She ate on the run, a chocolate, a snack from the checkout tills or a quick takeaway. Over the space of a year, she had gained five kilograms. She felt out of control. And the more out of control she felt, the more pedantic she became about minor details, the more perfectly she expected her children to behave and the more resentful she became of her husband, who she believed regarded her as just a housewife.

There were many aspects that Marilyn felt strongly about. Very early on in her journey of motherhood, she had made some clear choices about the way she wanted to show up as a mother. This was really important to her. But as her children grew up and needed her less, she felt justified in pursuing her passion. Over time, however, the clarity of what she wanted and what was important to her became blurred by the nitty gritty, practical aspects of managing a family, running a growing business, dealing with aging parents and a demanding extended family.

Naturally, Marilyn was the one everyone in her family came to when they wanted to host a fabulous birthday party, bachelorette party, baby shower, Christmas party or spring sundowners. They came to her because they knew she would do it well. They also knew she would never say no. And she never did; most of the time she loved watching a dream unfold into a fairytale event. The thought of saying no also left her with a gnawing guilt of letting them down, a fear of being judged. Many times she would chastise herself for taking on yet another project.

Eventually, she reached a point when she no longer had any capacity. She was exhausted, resentful and confused. She had had enough. She felt like running off to a place where no one could find her. The next best thing was to draw a line in the sand and start saying no. It was a Monday morning after her cousin's wedding, which she had helped organise. The kids were on holiday and she had a thousand things to arrange for the upcoming weekend's events. Her head was heavy and her body limp. She mustered up the energy to sit up and swing her legs over the edge of the bed, but collapsed back down again in a heap of despair. She knew that she needed help.

When I met Marilyn, her eyes bloodshot and heavy with accumulated tears and tiredness, she seemed burdened and anxious. She told a story of how nothing she was doing made sense anymore and wondered how a bubbly, passionate and self-aware person had spiraled down into such a dark place.

From boundaries to Boundfree

Marilyn's story was one that I hear over and over again in my practice. It is a story of those of us who start out with a clear vision, passion and energy. We are clear about what it is we want and know exactly what it takes to get there. With focus and determination, we move in the direction of our dreams. But somewhere along the journey, boundaries begin to blur, and energy gets compromised. In the quest of getting things done, we compromise on nourishing food, quality sleep, time with ourselves and for important relationships. Our lives get consumed with meeting deadlines, fulfilling demands and obligations and managing crises. When we are in the danger zone, we become confused about what we are actually responsible for and what we think we're responsible for. We vacillate between saying yes to everything and then saying no to everything when it all becomes too much. The reality is that neither end of the spectrum is useful in creating an energised life, and yet, the lack of boundaries to the creation of boundaries is an important step to arrive at a place that is Boundfree. A Boundfree response comes from a place of compassion and respect of self and others and that is in integrity with your value systems. It is not a rule-based boundary cast in stone, but rather has a flexible, responsive quality.

Very early on in our life experience we make an unconscious association between doing good and helping others, with being loved, appreciated and valued. It affirms our self-worth, gives our lives purpose and basically makes us feel good about who we are. Of course, this heart-centred way of living is wonderful and necessary. However, if we really had to examine our motivations deeply enough, we might see that what lurks in the shadow behind the well-intentioned and selfless 'doing good' is a fear of how we will be perceived, fear of disappointing others, guilt and conditioned thinking of what family and societal systems see as good and bad. Doing the right thing means that we toe the line, living according to societal norms. The alternative choice is judged selfish, narcissistic and self-serving.

Saying yes becomes a habit and pattern, even an addiction. A benchmark is created and we have successfully taught others how to treat us. We have officially become a dump yard, littered and cluttered with bullshit. But one day, something will stop you in your tracks; either some kind of realisation or some form of crisis, whether it is a health crisis, financial crisis, relationship breakdown or loss. It might take a few months to get to this place. Or a lifetime. You might get here early in your life without even knowing it. Or it might be a conscious choice you make later in your life. It can be a raw and frightening place to be because you feel exposed and vulnerable. Your self-preservation instinct kicks in. You retreat inwards. You draw the line in the sand. You start saying no. You create boundaries that you expect others to keep when dealing with you. You demand to be seen, to be heard, to be respected. You learn to start saying no and it feels good, it feels liberating.

It was at this point in Marilyn's journey that I met her. But her posture, her language and tone of voice did not reflect someone who had thrown off the shackles of responsibility. She seemed angry, bitter, confused and exhausted. Her boundary setting had started to work against her. People around her were confused by this sudden change in personality. They perceived her as distant and unapproachable, judgmental and condescending. Her boundary setting created conflict, which made her withdraw even further. She alienated her friends and sources of support. She felt isolated and alone.

For Marilyn, her energy management programme had to address the boundary issue as a priority. It was clear that this was at the root of her physical symptoms. Her need to set boundaries came from a place of resentment and vulnerability, and the need to protect herself from what she was feeling. When we set boundaries, we need to be very clear about the place from which we are setting them. Is it fuelled by anger? Is it an excuse to cop out and not take responsibility? When boundaries are too rigid or used as a defensive strategy, there is no flow. And we can close ourselves off to other possibilities and choices. Thus, there is a risk that boundaries are limiting and even more draining. In saying all of this, creating a boundary may be a crucial step on the journey of living with authentic energy, especially when we can bring awareness to the choices that we are making.

When we can make choices that are in alignment with our value system and that come from a place of intact self-worth, self-respect and disconnected from the fear of making those choices, then we are Boundfree.

Boundfree is not a line drawn in the sand, not a binary 'either or' generic rule. It is a dynamic process, a choice that is made in the moment and may be unique for a particular situation. A no today might be a yes tomorrow, depending on the situation, energy capacity and people involved. Boundfree is a new paradigm in boundaries. It is free from fear, guilt and resentment. It is a choice that is congruent with your value system and that is honouring of what you need in that moment. It is a responsive process that comes from a place of empathy, of compassion and respect for yourself and others. It's giving, sharing and helping in a way that does not compromise your own energy, happiness and health.

When you can do this, you free up energy to focus on what is really important to you and to direct awareness inwards.

Steps to becoming Boundfree in a particular situation

Ask yourself:
- What would your default response be to this situation?
- What impact would that decision have on your energy right now or in this particular situation?
- What is behind that pattern? Where does that come from? How did that pattern develop?
- What do you get from it? What is the payback for you? (This process requires stark honesty.)
- What are you compromising or giving up in the process?
- With this awareness, has your decision changed?
- Why? What would be the motivation for a different decision?
- How does this decision make you feel?
- How can you communicate this decision in a way that is clear using mindful language that does not make excuses to justify your choice to others, and is kind and compassionate to yourself and the other?

> Energy Formula
> *(Respect + compassion for yourself)* x *(respect and compassion for the other) - fear - resentment = authentic energy*

CHAPTER 16

Creating an energised life

When we can live from the heart, with curiosity and wonder, we can be inspired by anything and feel joy and freedom in expressing it.

> **LINDA'S STORY: ARCHITECTURE AND ALCHEMY**
> **Name:** Linda Naidoo
> **Age:** 41
> **Character traits:** Faith, fear
> **Life-changing experiences:** Twin sister's death
> **Stress catalysts in the last two years:** Work pressure
> **Stress indicators:** Chest pain, fainting spells (vasovagal attacks)
> **Presentation on energy zone map:** Burnout zone

Part 1

Every year in May when the trees stood half naked and the crunch of brown leaves were felt under feet, Linda would feel the same ache in her heart. From the way that the sun hung lower in the sky and cast longer shadows, to the feeling of the cool autumn air in her nostrils, every nuance of nature was a cruel reminder of the day that a big part of her also died.

Every year, a few days before the anniversary of her twin sister's tragic death, Linda would begin to feel the familiar rippling tension across her left shoulder, which culminated in a breathless spasm in her chest. Even after five years since that tragic accident, it still felt too big to metabolise. Work became her anaesthetic. It was familiar, safe and predictable in the way she needed it to be. It also helped to have a group of adventurous friends who dragged her along on hikes, picnics and weekends in the mountains. Linda loved the outdoors. Somehow, nature's balm felt more comforting than daily distractions. The grief strategy worked for a while. She was more than just functional at work. In fact, she thrived and got promoted to senior manager. Her IT skills were sought after, her expertise was valued and well rewarded both verbally and financially. Then one day, when her company won a major client and her boss held her in a congratulatory embrace, Linda unexpectedly broke down in tears. It flooded up, uncontainable and devastating. To her boss, her emotional reaction was confusing. Up to that point, she had made a conscious choice to keep a wide space between work and personal life, but that day she realised that she was a pressure cooker of grief and sadness, waiting to explode.

After five years, Linda knew she had to face her loss. She had just experienced the first glimpse of the alternative and it terrified her. Reluctantly, an appointment was made with a psychologist and every month for a year, through bite-sized chunks, she began to digest the enormity of her loss. Her therapy became more than a place to process her grief. The sessions provided the opportunity to dissect work dynamics and vent family frustrations. It created the space to bring awareness to the difference between her constructed external reality, which was capable, confident and in control, versus her inner world that felt so fractured. Linda felt deeply supported by her therapist and valued having the safe space to process her thoughts and feelings. But with mounting pressure at work, sitting on the therapy couch began to feel like an indulgence. She started to cancel more and more sessions and eventually stopped going all together. Work surreptitiously seeped into her down time, nature time, meal time and dream time, until there was nothing else. She stopped seeing her friends and memories of her sister got packed away like the box of photographs at the back of her cupboard.

One day, after a particularly long client meeting, Linda collapsed in the car park. They diagnosed a vasovagal attack (an overstimulated vagus nerve response causing a sharp drop in blood pressure, often attributed to shock or severe stress). Her family GP ran some tests, which revealed anaemia with low iron stores, and after thorough inquiry she suggested that she consider taking anti-depressants. Linda preferred to try a more conservative approach and that was when she called me.

When I met Linda, I was struck by her sense of easy style, her earthy-meets-urban-funk dress sense, her long dark curls and a wide smile that broke through her fatigue. When she relayed her story to me, through sobs and smiles, I cried with her. I realised how much the grief had taken its toll on her health and how the pressures at work had depleted her energy resources. Linda had all the classic signs of vital exhaustion; she ticked every box of the burnout zone on the energy zone map both physically and psychologically. Her blood tests confirmed that her adrenal glands were taking strain. Her cortisol levels had dropped as had her DHEA, the mother hormone that feeds the production for both cortisol and progesterone, which also helped to explain her PMS symptoms. Her brittle nails and dry skin told me a story of real nutritional deficiencies, which I was sure was adding to her low mood. While her muscle tension was high, her blood pressure was low. Linda was also underweight for her height. We needed to address Linda's physical health as a matter of urgency.

And so we began the journey of putting the basics in place. We crafted an eating plan that felt practical to plan, shop for and prepare. Using the Mediterranean diet as a basis, we added some herbs and spices to appeal to her finely developed Indian palate and that supported her body type. I prescribed a range of supplements, which included adaptogenic herbs to nourish the adrenal glands and some that addressed the anaemia. We were building her foundation of health again, waking up her body intelligence and supporting her emotional health at the same time.

After three months of working intensively to restore Linda's physical health, she felt ready to revisit the trauma of her sister's death. While her initial psychotherapy had supported her to make sense of her grief process, her body was still holding it on a cellular level. Each time she thought about her sister and the events that led to the tragedy, she felt the trigger spot of tension threatening to activate the spasm. She couldn't deny the connection. But even this awareness did little to quell her deepening anxiety that there was more to this pain, that it was more serious, more ominous and life threatening. And as much as medical investigations have the capacity to do, we ruled out any probability of this.

Linda needed to re-establish her sense of trust in her body, and rather than reacting to her symptoms, she needed to respond to them with a broader perspective using the principles of recovery loops, body intelligence, mind intelligence and heart intelligence.

Conscious breathing became one of the key techniques that Linda felt was simple and practical to apply. Each time she felt physical tension, she learned to breathe in to soften up the muscles rather than tense up even more. Taking small steps, Linda began to trust her body again, knowing that if she took care of the basic pillars, her IPOL would kick in and her body would function in the way it was designed. She practised using the breath as recovery loops to break the cycle of adrenalised energy during the day and used a different technique to help her fall asleep at night. She also used her breathing to dive into and channel her feelings rather than building a wall around them. Then one day something wonderful happened. Linda walked into my room, sparkly eyed, hair tied up in a messy bun. She came bearing a gift. The excited unwrapping revealed a small square canvas on which was the most compelling piece of art, abstract and vague, yet the strokes and blending of colours told a poignant story of sadness and joy, healing and hope.

Her gift to me was also a commitment to herself, a new

beginning. She had re-ignited a childhood passion for art and now she was using it in a different way. Grief, burnout and physical exhaustion had stripped away all the layers of her constructed identity, leaving her raw and exposed like the trees in May. Her job title, her possessions, her body, she felt like she had lost it all or that it meant nothing. And in that rawness, that trembling fearful place, she released her grip and fell into her own depth, her essence, her heart. In doing so she accessed the richness of what it contained; her passion, her creativity, hope, trust, energy. Now all she needed was to construct a new scaffolding through which to express it.

Part 2

One year later
She was warned that it was going to be a tough session but she was ready. Light protein breakfast, a good 20-minute warm up and she was good to go. Linda positioned her feet, bent her knees into a squat, gripped the bar, and with all the power of breath, body and will lifted 30 kilograms off the ground.

The day that Linda brought me the painting was the day that she committed to designing a new life, with a clear intention and focus, aligned with her values and yet open to the possibilities of a life that she could perhaps not yet envision. She experienced first-hand how she was able to access her inner resources to heal and work through her grief. Now she was ready to use this energy to flourish, grow and create the life she knew she was worthy of and deserved. No longer did she carry the guilt that she should have been the one who died that day instead of her sister. Nor did she feel torn between the corporate world and creative dreams. She wanted both. Needed both. Of course, this didn't mean that she didn't experience moments of sheer terror about her future or doubt about her choices. But these moments came and passed quickly, feelings became like passing clouds. She knew what peace felt like. And so she created more and more opportunities to feel it. She knew her Stillpoint and the moments in time that filtered out the noise to take her there. Nature, art, creative spaces and conversations opened her heart and gave her the energy to carry her forward. She blended the art of science of her body and being to be the architect of her life. Her own alchemist.

In one of her sessions we sat together and wrote the story of her future self; the life she desired to live, how she wanted to feel, and the kind of life that supported both this feeling and her values. She wrote it as if it was happening, as if it was real, down to the last detail. It was far more challenging than she had anticipated. She became aware of all her old beliefs of why it couldn't happen, old emotional patterning that she felt she didn't deserve it, and judgements of how far her life felt from that dream. After filtering out the fear, we distilled her clear intention for an energised, abundant and fulfilling life, anchored to stillness and able to surf the waves of life.

The story Linda wrote about her future life told of one who shared her life with a partner who supported her to be the best she could be, a fulfilling career that allowed her to use her skills and that allowed the financial freedom and flexibility to pursue her creative pursuits, whether it be through hobbies or creative business. While not fixated on having a child, she was open to the possibility. Definitely not more than one though. A pet was part of the picture, a dog with floppy ears. A cozy home with an open plan living area, lots of light, vegetable patch, creative space and the sound of running water. Adventure travel at least every two years. Machu Pichu, Kilimanjaro, Camino de Compostela, skiing in Patagonia, trekking in Bhutan. Meaningful time with people that mattered, quiet time for herself to reflect and connect. Giving back in some way. Time in nature. A daily routine, nourishing delicious food. Trust in life. A strong, flexible body. A calm and focused mind and a wide open heart.

She wrote it all down, every last detail, even if it felt clichéd. It is what SHE wanted and committed to creating. Not in a fixated, controlled way, but in an open-minded and intentional way. Yes, she had experienced some deep pain, loss and tragedy in her life and, of course, she knew that life would present more loss and adversity. But this time she wanted to have the best shot at facing it, feeling it and growing from it. Burnout had shown her that it was possible.

Every three months, or whenever Linda was faced with a choice or given an opportunity, she would take out her page and be reminded of what she was creating.

At the time of writing, Linda had slowly and steadily built up her strength, flexibility and fitness to a point where she can lift a 30 kg barbell. This was not just about the physical strength, though, it was a moment when her belief in herself, and her focus and commitment culminated and worked together in a magnificent way. The way she was able to open to her breath, lock in her core strength, and harness her energy was thrilling.

Linda is becoming a master of her energy; she knows what adrenalised energy feels like, when it's not appropriate and how to discharge it. She also knows how to use it and how to recover and replenish afterwards. She has trained recovery loops into her daily routine and on most days feels energised. On other days, she takes it easy and slows down the pace as much as possible. She has adopted a loveable puppy and spends weekends in front of big canvases, in denim dungarees and messy overalls. Each time she goes back to read the vision she crafted that day, she is amazed by how much closer she is getting to creating it, through her conscious choices, effort and the mystery of what she can't see but knows is there. The partner hasn't shown up yet, but I have a feeling that he's hovering around. It's been a wonderful inspiring privilege to witness Linda's journey and so many others who have made a commitment to living their best life.

Staying authentically energised

Each day I sit in awe and fascination at our capacity to create an inspired life and how often adversity can become grist for the mill. When we are able to trust magic, the unknown and stay grounded and practical at the same time, we are able to express authentic energy in the most surprising ways. Creative energy challenges mediocrity, demands individuality, and provokes mob mentality. Maybe that's why we are here. We are creations ourselves and we have a responsibility to continuously contribute to the process of creativity. We have an instinct to create and challenge stale and automated lives. When we can live from the heart, with curiosity and wonder, we can be inspired by anything and feel joy and freedom in expressing that, whether it be through the way we dress, how we walk across a room, how we set the table or put a meal together. It may come through as inspiration for a new strategy at work or an idea for a business. It could be expressed in the way we put words together in an email or through a wacky sense of humour. For some, it may come in the form of a specific talent. But for all of us it is about using it to create a life that we truly want and deserve.

When we are tired, burnt out and disillusioned, we become disconnected from this inspiration or source energy. And the more disconnected we are, the more empty we feel. The more we dip into source energy, through the body, mind and heart, the more we can start to see new possibilities for our life.

When we do open up to the energy of creativity, we have a responsibility to it and ourselves to use it consciously. If untamed, the creative force becomes like wild fire, rampant and devastating to the physical form through which it is expressed. We have to support and respect the body as the vehicle for the creative force. We come across too many talented, creative souls who throw the fuelled adrenalised energy to the creative fire. This can be dangerous for those who do not replenish their physical and emotional resources.

I'm constantly blown away by our human capacity to create works of art, buildings and inventions, tools for nanotechnology, and spaceships that propel us into the universe itself. What is even more magnificent is our ability to create a new life, our ability to heal, create fresh architecture in our brain and bodies. I see the magnificence of this process every single day, I see it in

Linda's story, Nidara's story, Felix's story, Leo's story, my story. With commitment, intention, focus, perseverance, support and courage, we move slowly to mold, chisel and constantly work on the creation of our lives.

Using the energy formulas

We are now ready to craft a journey using all the energy formulas that we have formulated to design a brand new body–mind system. Fresh neural pathways will be laid, health-promoting genes will be unregulated as your cells wake up. The new architecture will support the flow of authentic, creative energy. When you align this energy with your intention, life will begin to move in the direction of your dreams. This doesn't mean that you will not face adversity and pain, it means that you will be able to use it as material and inspiration for your new life.

Get out some paper, make some tea, and make some time for this process:

Step 1
Plot yourself on the energy zone map. Name the current circumstances of your life that you believe are causing you to be in this place.

Step 2
What aspects of this life work for you? In other words, list the aspects of your life that are important for you to hold onto and nurture. What is not working and that you would like to release or let go of? Why? What aspects of your life need an adjustment?

Step 3
In as much detail as you can, describe the life that you would like to live. Describe your home, what you spend your days doing, how you make a living, where you travel, who you spend time with, how you relax, what your recovery loops look like. This should

include everything that gives you energy.

Examine what is behind each of those times you describe. Why do believe it's important?

Step 4

What source of energy do you believe needs the most support right now? Body, mind or heart intelligence? Choose one.

One of my teachers, Bernard Brom, reminds his students that we don't need to plug all the holes. We are an interconnected system of body, mind, heart and energy. Even if we put one thing in place, IPOL will wake up to support the other sources.

Choose one energy formula you would like to work with. Commit to practising this energy formula for 40 days. Journal your thoughts, insights and experiences for 40 days. Revisit the energy zone map.

> Energy Formula
> *Apply one energy formula + intention = authentic energy*
> Authentic energy is your right. The world is waiting.

CHAPTER 17

Our story: Thanksgiving

> *Gratitude has the ability to shift our perspective on anything that is causing pain, irritation or frustration.*

We are drowning in adrenaline. We have become seduced by the material benefits of hard work. The systems in which we live and work reward being busy, tired and frenetic as if it's a measure of success. The idea of 'burning out' is becoming an accepted and expected narrative in our society. Even if we are driven by passion and purpose, unless we tap into authentic energy, we get tired. We burn out. And when we burn out, we stop caring – for ourselves and others. We disconnect from our humanity. We are seeing the devastating effects of this disconnection everywhere. Authentic energy is our natural state and our birthright. We have a responsibility to ourselves and future generations to access it and to find meaningful ways to connect with ourselves, each other and nature.

Breathe has been written to explore ways to tap into this energy by attending to our bodies, the vehicle for our consciousness, by taking responsibility for the way we think, our choices and behaviours and by tuning in to our feelings, emotions and the wisdom of our hearts. We can't always get it right, but by developing a more honest and meaningful relationship with ourselves we can reach into the world from a more whole and authentic place. We can be real about how and when to be busy and adrenalised and we can have the awareness and courage to stop and turn inwards and rest and replenish and see the world through grateful eyes again.

I believe that gratitude must be the highest form of heart intelligence. Thousands of studies have been done on it now, proving the link between deep genuine gratitude to happiness, empathy, reduced aggression, self-esteem, sleep, resilience. We even have gratitude researchers who dedicate their lives to this work, with The Institute of HeartMath in the US. While the research is compelling, do we really need studies to tell us how gratitude makes us feel?

The other day I was 'free writing' my thoughts on gratitude and everything in my life that inspires gratitude. I was amazed and surprised. I particularly challenged myself to feel gratitude for the situations that I'm angry or frustrated about. As I was going through the exercise, I literally felt the shift in my energy. It was a beautiful feeling of lightness and expansion that I carried all day. The state of gratitude brought me more deeply into every moment, kept me present and made me feel grateful for everything!

Gratitude has the ability to shift our perspective on anything that is causing pain, irritation or frustration. It heightens heart intelligence, sharpens mind intelligence and supports body intelligence. Gratitude reminds us of our natural state, which is peaceful and free.

I don't have an energy formula for gratitude. I think it stands on its own. Add a deep breath and gratitude to every energy formula you use and I think you'll have a winning formula for a healthy, inspired and authentically energised life.

Acknowledgements

To Natasha Frachiolla, the angel of words and magic maker, soul sister and writing coach, words do not suffice to express my gratitude. Your belief in me and skill in the craft of writing is one of the big reasons that this work came into being. A massive thank you to Marj Murray, who stood by me every step of the way in the process of birthing this book and who spent hours over the drafts seeing what I couldn't on more than one level. I'm infinitely grateful to Marj for being my voice of reason, steadfast supporter and amazing friend. I bow in deep gratitude to Marisa Farinha Lloyd, whose voice and heart is so intimately woven into this book and who constantly nudges me to the edge of my comfort zone. I am eternally grateful to Dan Brulé for his unconditional support, friendship, mentorship and love. To Dorian and Leigh Cabral, my trainers and friends who support my authentic energy and who've helped me to not just lift the ceiling but remove it, thank you.

Hament Nagar, my husband, my rock and best friend, inspires and supports me in ways he will never know. He makes what I do possible and easy. I am blessed to share a life with someone who is a true example of authentic energy and integrity. To Hament, your love, support and patience with me means everything. Thank you.

To my publisher Melinda Ferguson, thank you for believing in me and the purpose of this book.

To the team at Jacana Media, a big thanks to you.

This book was shaped by the deeply moving stories of people I have had the privilege of sitting with in my consultation room every day. Your healing and growth is my healing and growth. I have lived each chapter with you. And I am so enriched because of it.

I have a truly beautiful and blessed life, mostly because it is touched by special friends, who have become my soul family. Our conversations and mingled paths are all part of this book. You know who you are. Deep gratitude to you.

And finally, gratitude to you, dear reader.

Glossary of terms

Adrenalised energy: The high energy state that is felt in response to stress, whether real or perceived. While adrenalised energy is necessary to life, it becomes harmful when prolonged and not balanced by rest and recovery.

Authentic energy: The vibrant centred quality of energy that is fueled by source energy (natural energy) and is expressed through the body, mind and heart. It occurs when one lives in tune with nature's rhythms and cycles and when the sympathetic (high-energy stress response) is balanced with the parasympathetic (rest and recovery mode).

Ayurveda: Translated as the 'Science of Life', it is an ancient system of living originating in India 5000 years ago. It honours the interconnectedness of the mind–body system and our connection with nature. It offers guidance on all aspects of natural living and managing energy based on our unique body types.

Body intelligence: The optimum functioning of the human body as a vehicle and expression of source energy. It is directed by IPOL and is experienced when we support its basics needs.

Boundfree: A choice that is made from a place that is compassionate and respectful of self and others that is in integrity with your value systems. It is not a rule-based boundary cast in stone, but rather has a flexible, responsive quality.

Glossary of terms

Burnout zone: A chronic state of depletion of authentic energy that manifests physically, emotionally, behaviourally and spiritually.

Danger zone: A set of physical and behavioural symptoms that indicate that an individual is starting to experience the harmful effects of adrenalised energy.

Doshas: Primary life forces or 'humors' are derived from the five elements and are responsible for the physical and psychological functions of our body. According to Ayurveda, each individual has a combination of all three doshas of Pitta, Vata and Kapha with a predominance of one or two that we are born with, and one which predominates at any particular time. Understanding your type or what is out of balance is helpful in assisting in adjusting lifestyle choices and staying in the optimum zone. Many of us show a combination of dosha types.

- Pitta (Fire): Characteristics include being of medium, athletic build and well proportioned. They are dynamic, ambitious, competitive and passionate. They feel hot and sensitive, emotionally and physically. Balancing Pitta requires cooling foods, avoidance of extreme exercise and calming activities.
- Vata (Wind): Usually slim and small boned. They feel cold easily and tend to have dry skin. They are often highly creative, restless, unpredictable and energetic, but tire easily. They require grounding stability and routine to keep them centred and prefer warm and humid environments to keep their system in balance.
- Kapha (Earth): Kapha types have a larger build and tend to put on weight easily due to a slow metabolism. They are strong, resilient, grounded, calm and routine orientated. They do best with activities that boost heat and fuel a faster metabolism, such as smaller, more frequent meals and stimulating forms of exercise.

Energy zone map: A map that illustrates a typical pattern of energy as it gets depleted and lists the physical, behavioural and emotional symptoms as one progresses from optimum zone to danger zone and finally to burnout zone.

Heart intelligence: The wisdom and energy that we experience when are deeply connected to ourselves and our feelings, to others and to nature.

IPOL or intelligent pulse of life: The innate intelligent force that resides within every living organism that directs healing, growth, adaptation and evolutionary processes.

Mind intelligence: The ability of the mind to optimise energy through focus, concentration and self-awareness and to be a channel for source energy through creativity, innovative thinking and inspiration.

Optimum zone: An emotional and physical state of being that is reflective of living with optimised authentic energy.

Recovery loop: A conscious activation of the parasympathetic nervous system that taps into natural energy resources through the body, mind or heart, or all three. It could also be any activity that brings a sense of calm, peace and wellbeing, giving the body, mind and soul time to recover from long periods of stress and intensity. A recovery loop can range from one second (micro recovery loop) like a yawn, sigh or stretch, to a walk in the park or a long weekend away (macro recovery loop).

Source energy: Life force or natural energy that we are an expression of.

Stillpoint: A moment in time when the noise of everyday life is filtered out and a state deep peace, joy and wellbeing is felt, and authentic energy can be accessed.

References

Adams, C. 2012. *Breathing to Heal: The Science of Healthy Respiration*. Logical Books, Wilmington, Delaware.

Aserinsky, E & Kleitman N. 1953. Regularly occurring periods of eye motility, concomitant phenomena, during sleep. *Science*, 118 (3062): 273–274.

Ballantine, R. 1990. *Radical Healing: Integrating the World's Great Therapeutic Traditions to Create a New Transformative Medicine*. Harmony Books, New York.

Brown, B. 2012. *Daring Greatly*. Random House, New York.

Breathnach, S B. 2002. *Romancing the Ordinary: A Year of Simple Splendour*. Jenson Books Inc., Both Logan, Utah.

Bhasin, M K, Dusek, J A, Chang, B H, Joseph, M G, Denninger, J W, Fricchione, G L, Benson, H, Libermann, T A. 2013. Relaxation response induces temporal transcriptome changes in energy metabolism, insulin secretion and inflammatory pathways. *PLoS One* 8(5).

Brulé, D. *Shut Up and Breathe*. Available at www.breathmastery.com (accessed 25 May 2014).

Brulé, D. 2017. *Just Breathe*. Simon and Schuster, New York.

Chopra, D. 1989. *Quantum Healing: Exploring the Frontiers of Mind Body Medicine*. Bantam Books, New York.

Chopra, D. 1990. *Perfect Health: The Complete Mind Body Guide*. Harmony Books, New York.

Cameron, J. 1993. *The Artists Way.* Pan Books, United Kingdom.

Dispenza, J. 2007. *Evolving your Brain: The Science of Changing your Mind.* Health Communications Inc., Florida.

Dispenza, J. 2012. *Breaking the Habit of Being Yourself, How to Lose Your Mind and Create a New One.* Hay House, California.

Davidson, R J & Begley, S. 2012 *The Emotional Life of Your Brain.* Plume, Penguin Group, London.

Doige, N. 2007. *The Brain that Changes Itself.* Penguin Books, London.

Durham, N C, Pieper, C, Philips-Bute, B, Bryant, J & Kuhn, C. 2002. Caffeine's effects are long lasting and compound stress. *Duke Medicine News and Communications,* 64(4):595–603.

Fried, R. 1999. *Breathe Well, Be Well: A Program to Relieve Stress, Anxiety, Asthma, Hypertension, Migraine, and Other Disorders for Better Health.* John Wiley and Sons, New York.

Grandner, M A, Gallagher, R A L & Gooneratne, N S. 2013. The use of technology at night: Impact on sleep and health. *Sleep Med* 9(12):1301–1302.

Goleman, D. 1995. *Emotional Intelligence.* Bloomsbury Publishing, New York.

Haas, Elson. 2003. *Keeping Healthy with the Seasons.* Celestial Arts, California.

Hansen, R & Medius, R. 2009. *Buddha's Brain: The Neuroscience of Happiness, Love and Wisdom.* New Harbinger Publications Inc., California.

Iber Ancoli-Israel, S, Chesson, A L & Quan, S F. 2007. The AASM manual for the scoring of sleep and associated events: Rules, terminology and technical specification. *Journal of Clinical Sleep Medicine* 13(4): 597–619.

Iyengar, B K S. 1981. *Light on Pranayama.* Harper Collins, New York

Juliano, L M & Griffiths, R R. 2005. 'Caffeine', in Lowinson, J H, Ruiz, P, Millman, R B, Langrod, J G (eds.) *Substance Abuse: A Comprehensive Textbook, Fourth Edition.* Lippincott, Williams & Wilkins. Baltimore.

Kabat-Zinn, J. 1990. *Full Catastrophe Living: How to Cope with Stress, Pain and Illness Using Mindfulness Meditation.* Bantam Books, New York.

Katie, B. 2008. *Who Would You Be Without Your Story?* Hay House, California.

Kahneman, D. 2011. *Thinking Fast and Slow.* Penguin Books, London.

Lazar, S W, Kerr, C E, Wasserman, R H, Gray, J R, Greye, D N, Treadway, M T, McGarvey, M, Quinn, B T, Dusek, J A, Benson, H, Rauch, S L, Moore, C I, Fischl, Bruce. 2005. 'Meditation experience is associated with increased cortical thickness', *Neuroport* 16(17):1893–1897.

Lewis, D. 2004. *Free your Breath, Free your Life.* Shambhala Publications, Colorado.

Levitin, D. 2014. *The Organised Mind. Thinking Straight in the Age of Information Overload.* Penguin Books, New York.

Lipton, B H. 2005. *Biology of Belief: Unleashing the Power of Consciousness Matter and Miracles.* Mountain of Love/Elite Books, Santa Rosa.

Manga, E. 2016. *Burnout to Breathing.* Available at: www.drelamanga.com (accessed on 18 October 2016).

McCraty, R. 2015. Heart–brain neurodynamics: The making of emotions in issues of the heart. In Dahlitz, M & Hall, G (eds) *Issues of the Heart: The Neuropsychotherapist.* Special Issue. Dahlitz Media: Brisbane, pp. 76–110.

McIntyre, A. 2012. *The Ayurveda Bible. The Definitive Guide to Ayurvedic Healing.* Octopus Publishing Group, London.

O'Hare, D. 2014. *Heart Coherence 365. A Guide to Long-lasting Heart Coherence.* Thierry Salccar Editions, France.

Pert, C. 1997. *Molecules of Emotion: Why You Feel the Way You Feel.* Simon and Schuster, New York.

Peckham, C. 2015. *Physician burnout: It just keeps getting worse.* Available at: www.medscape.com/viewarticle/838437 (accessed on 15 April 2015).

Rama, S, Ballantine, R & Hymes, A. 1979: *Science of Breath: A Practical Guide.* Himalayan Institute Press, Pennsylvania.

Rosen, L. 2012. *iDisorder. Understanding Our Obsession with Technology and Overcoming Its Hold on Us.* Palgrave Macmillan, London.

Scharmer, O & Kaufer, K. 2013. *Leading from the Emerging Future: From Ego-System to Eco-System Economies.* Berrett-Koehler Publishers, California.

Scharmer, O. 2009. *Theory U: Leading from the Future as it Emerges.* Berrett-Koehler Publishers, California.

Scott, S J. 2016. *Habit Stacking: 97 Small Life Changes that Take 5*

Minutes or Less. Oldtown Publishing LLC, New Jersey.
Tolle, E. 1999. *The Power of Now*. New World Library, San Francisco.
Tolle, E, 2006, *Stillness Amidst the World*. New World Library, San Francisco.

Other useful websites

www.HeartMath.org
www.laughteryoga.org
www.susangreenfield.com

www.ingramcontent.com/pod-product-compliance
Lightning Source LLC
Chambersburg PA
CBHW071353290426
44108CB00014B/1536